the BEST DIET *on* EARTH

ORDINARY FOODS WITH EXTRAORDINARY POWERS

based on the DASH DIET

by **Linda Levy** and
Francine Grabowski, MS, RD, CDE

LAKE ISLE PRESS, INC. / NEW YORK

Published by Lake Isle Press, Inc.
16 West 32nd St., Suite 10-B
New York, NY 10001
lakeisle@earthlink.net

Distributed to the trade by:
National Book Network (NBN), Inc.
4720 Boston Way
Lanham, MD 20706
1(800)462-6420
http://www.nbnbooks.com

Library of Congress Control Number: 2003190002
ISBN: 1-891105-08-6

Small portions of this book, including several recipes, previously appeared
in LOW-FAT LIVING FOR REAL PEOPLE, 2nd ed., by Linda Levy and Francine Grabowski, MS, RD,
published by Lake Isle Press, Inc. (1998).

Cover photos: Paul Levy
Thanks to Don Rellstab, Pennington Quality Market, for the "photo op."

Book and cover design: Chris Kalb

This book is available at special sales discounts for bulk purchases
as premiums or special editions, including personalized covers.
For more information, contact the publisher: (212)273-0796 or by e-mail.

10 9 8 7 6 5 4 3 2 1

DEDICATION

For our grandchildren —
Charlie, Eli, and Cate
Jacqueline, Dryden, and Madeleine

TABLE OF CONTENTS

ACKNOWLEDGMENTS

WE THANK THE DASH RESEARCHERS, who proved that Mother Nature does indeed know best; the many people we have met who have had the courage to make changes for better health; M.Kyu Chung, who heads the Department of Family Medicine at Cooper Health Systems, and who welcomes and values a nutritional approach to health care; and Angela Shaw, who supports and teaches and lives the healthy way. We thank our playful and creative book designer, Chris Kalb. And we thank our publisher, Hiroko Kiiffner, whose gifts of wisdom and humor are a joy for us.

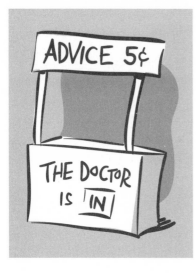

MEET THE EXPERT

Francine Grabowski, one of the authors of this book, has, among other letters after her name, R.D. An R.D. — "registered dietitian" — has extensive training and experience in helping people choose food for better health. Grabowski has worked with thousands of people over the past twenty years; you could call her "experienced." These people have helped her come to realize how important food is, and that choosing food for health is the best way to start taking care of yourself. She is inspired to do what she does, every day, and she loves doing it. As Grabowski says, "You know what? It's fun!" ★ So if you've never visited a registered dietitian, and didn't know what one is, now you do. ★ If you haven't been successful with food/lifestyle changes or weight issues, you need help, plain and simple. What follows are words of wisdom from our co-author and resident dietitian, Francine Grabowski. She is about to tell you some of her real-life experiences with patients, patients with real-life problems. She is an inspiration to them.

Obviously, this book can't take the place of a visit to a dietitian, but, as the old telephone company ads used to say, "It's the next best thing to being there." Read on about a way of eating that has been shown to lower blood pressure, a wonderful diet called "DASH." Read on about a way of eating that will decrease your risk of heart disease, cancer, diabetes. DASH and more! Read on about a way to eat not only for health, but also to be a healthy weight. It's all here: THE BEST DIET ON EARTH.

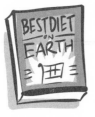

Francine Grabowski:

"SO WHAT ARE YOU GOING TO NAME THE BOOK?" asked a dear colleague from North Jersey when she heard about the project. When I said, *"THE BEST DIET ON EARTH,"* her immediate response was, "The DASH diet *is* the best diet on earth." And then we excitedly talked about our experiences with DASH.

Let me begin with my favorite story, about the 46-year-old woman with two children in grade school who attended one of my classes. She made it clear that she ate poorly: no breakfast, no fruit, no vegetables, no milk. She had had high blood pressure for three years, and her doctor warned her that she would need additional medication because the pressure was so poorly controlled. I was convinced there was a connection between her high blood pressure and her food choices. Well, she began to make changes. She followed the DASH diet, *and within a few short weeks, she was able to lower her blood pressure enough to get off her medications!* But she did a lot more than lower her blood pressure. When I called to find out how she was doing, she told me ecstatically, "I've lost weight, I have more energy. My husband doesn't know what's come over me." Her final comment? "It's so easy!"

Now let's talk about you, because, finally, this book is for you. It's about how you can make changes in order to take care of yourself. I promise you will feel an enormous sense of pride, pleasure, and accomplishment when you begin to make those changes.

I want you to be successful, and you are reading the right book to help you be successful! In my twenty years of working with patients, I've seen which patterns lead to success and which do not.

So what does it take? In a word, readiness. I am here now to help you decide if you are really ready to make the kinds of changes that will improve your health and your life.

Now — are you ready to do this? Are you? Good! Here we go —

THE FIRST STEP

IT ALL STARTS WITH A PHONE CALL. Maybe your doctor has been telling you to call for years, and finally you do that. Making that phone call is your first step in a commitment to change, which is hard work. I know and you know that this phone call is not about giving up cupcakes and pizza. It's about examining a whole life and making a decision to take care of yourself. Just know that you and I are joining forces in this.

The first thing we need to do together is check the road for obstacles, stumbling blocks that may, just may, get in your way. Simply being aware of them helps you to move forward.

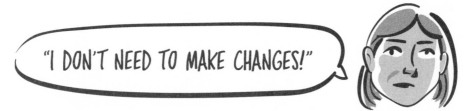

"I DON'T NEED TO MAKE CHANGES!"

Maybe you begin your visit to me with the words, "I've had high blood pressure and high cholesterol for 25 years and nothing has ever happened to me."

What you are really saying is, "Why should I change now?" Your experience has shown you that you are indestructible, an armored tank. No health condition can stop you. But wait! Why are you here? Something or somebody has convinced you to take a long, hard look at your health. Something or somebody is concerned that your days of being an armored tank may be numbered.

It's a good thing you're here, even if you don't think you need to make changes just yet. Let's hope you can continue to be an armored tank. But just to be on the safe side, stick around, read the book, and let's look at some other options.

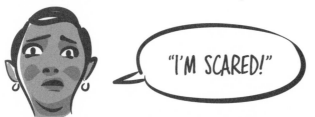

"I'M SCARED!"

When Carla doesn't show up for her second appointment, I remember something she said during her first visit. "Ten years ago, I took care of my mother when she had a stroke. I can't believe I'm here with the same health problems my mother had before she got sick!"

It takes courage to schedule that visit with me, to commit to change. You might find that your health problems are making you sad and scared, that these problems remind you of experiences you have had with a loved one.

However, you may well take a different path, which is why you've come to see me. Medical science has changed, with new and better treatments. Not only that, you have a greater awareness of what needs to be done to take care of yourself. Call it a competitive edge. You know what's in the family genes, so you can be prepared. This is about taking care of yourself, and if you're not doing that, it might help to explore these issues with a therapist.

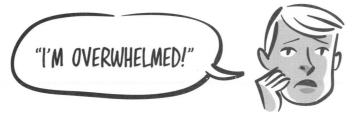

John, a 63-year-old retired manager of computer operations, comes into the office with these words: "I've been healthy all my life and now everything is wrong with me. I have a doctor's appointment almost daily. I don't know what to do or where to start."

Too much change at any one time can be overwhelming. It certainly is unfair that just at the time you are supposed to be living out the dreams you made when you planned for this retirement, you are spending time at medical appointments — in fact, more medical appointments in the past six months than in the last few years put together. Change can sometimes be thrust upon you when you are least expecting it. Bad timing and bad luck.

It is important for you to remember that this is a transition, and it will pass. It is annoying — maybe even heart-breaking — but it is a transition, and it will get easier. Make sure you surround yourself with caring people and healthcare workers who want to support you during this time.

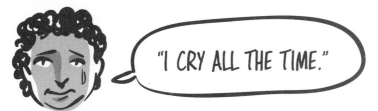

Sometimes a person comes to see me and within five minutes is crying, crying for everything — for all of life's miseries, and yet for nothing in particular. This is a person who is living a joyless life.

We all want to be happy. It's built in. No, it might not be 24 hours a day, but it's our right. If you find you aren't happy, that you are brought to tears easily, that you feel overwhelmed, maybe have trouble sleeping, then talk to your doctor. There could be a medical reason, perhaps a clinical depression. Or you might need to work with a therapist to sort out the patterns that lead to unhappiness.

Please, please look at the root of your unhappiness before embarking on nutrition changes. *Food does not solve the happiness problem. Losing weight will not bring you joy.* You will need your internal "spark of happiness" to be in good working order before you make changes in the way you eat.

> **"SORRY, BUT I JUST DON'T LIKE VEGETABLES."**

You say you're ready to make changes, but you have just one small issue: You've never eaten vegetables, even as a child. You say you cannot put a vegetable in your mouth no matter how hard you try.

You may think this is a small issue, but the truth is you have a handicap. If your inability to eat vegetables is that powerful, then you are in the ranks of the vegetable delayed. It will be almost impossible to make a change. The only answer is to consider giving vegetables another chance.

With any luck, there's a faint glimmer of hope that this is not a permanent situation. Terrific! Put it on your list of worthwhile goals. Join forces with that spouse or friend who has been urging you for years to eat vegetables. You might surprise yourself. Stranger things have happened.

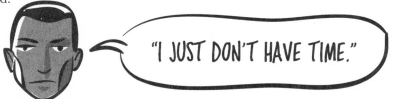

> **"I JUST DON'T HAVE TIME."**

Tom, a business executive in his 40's who suffers from heart disease, calls me up to cancel his appointment. He is very apologetic, explaining that his business is downsizing and he has to work longer hours. "I just don't have time," he says.

Not having "enough time" is the number one reason people cannot make changes in their lives. Time is a precious commodity — only 24 hours in each day at last count — and the way you use it reflects what you value. You must be convinced that keeping your appointment with your dietitian (or anyone else, for that matter) is important. If you don't think it is — well, you'll cancel it to make time for something that you think is more important.

What Tom is really saying to me when he cancels an appointment because he doesn't have time is, *"Making changes for my health is not a value in my life at this time."* It is very clear that work is the most important thing to him right now. I also know that he doesn't have time for family dinners or his daughter's soccer game.

So to the Toms everywhere, make sure you are spending your time on what really matters to you. Look around you and see what is really important. Now prove it is important by giving it time. Of course there are temporary time constraints that will always arise: a daughter's wedding, or the need to study for the bar. But if your time constraints last years, you might want to sit back and check to see if your time truly reflects your deepest values.

"I'VE BECOME A CAREGIVER WITH NO TIME FOR MYSELF."

On the other hand, this may not be the time to make changes. Mary is a high school principal who was successfully making changes until her father became ill. She visits him at the hospital every day, and then on weekends helps her mother with chores and bills. She has, of necessity, become a care-giver with physically demanding responsibilities as well as intense emotional day-to-day care.

If you have become such a caregiver, your own health may actually decline as you devote time to taking care of someone else. This is a good time to seek support for the extreme stress of your situation. Find a support group. Maybe your cousins, maybe your friends, maybe your church. But make sure you have a support group.

Give yourself a break. Recognize the little things you do every day that take care of YOU. In Mary's case, she discovered that she walks a lot in the course of a work day. It is far from one end of the building to the other, a distance she covers several times a day. Just knowing this brought her a quiet sense of accomplishment, and that felt good.

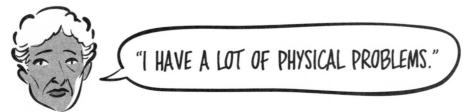

"I HAVE A LOT OF PHYSICAL PROBLEMS."

Sara is in a wheel chair and needs to make the kinds of changes that will allow her to lose weight. I explain to her that it will be difficult, as she has trouble moving around and cannot do the sort of exercise that generally helps people lose weight.

If you have serious physical limitations and can't move around very much, the chances are you will *gain* weight. Since losing weight will be particularly difficult for you, you will need to choose your foods very, very carefully. This is not easy. There are already many restrictions in your life, and now you are being told to restrict your food.

Even though you are in a wheelchair, you can still exercise. First, of course, talk to your doctor so you can figure out what kind of physical activity will work for you. Be prepared to call health clubs, the local hospital, and the community center in your area to locate facilities and personnel that can help you. You will be rewarded with community support.

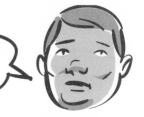

"NO MATTER HOW HARD I TRY, I CAN'T LOSE WEIGHT."

Robert comes into my office and begins his visit by saying, "I can't lose weight."

Lots of people come to me with this complaint. You may also have trouble losing weight. If so, your first job is to make an appointment with your doctor for a thorough medical examination. Discuss your concerns. Maybe there are medical reasons why you can't lose weight.

Lay The Groundwork For Successful Weight Loss

☞ Carve out time in your life to take care of yourself. (And be realistic about how much time you can carve out at this moment.)

☞ Demand excellent and thorough medical care.

☞ Trust that the work you are doing will make you feel healthier, give you more energy, and give you a sense of accomplishment.

Deciding to make lifestyle changes means you will commit a certain period of time to surrounding yourself with information and guidance in order to find the strategies that fit into your life. You have the ability to be creative and find ways to make changes. In her superb book "Thin for Life," Anne Fletcher interviewed 160 people who had made health changes to lose weight, calling them "masters of weight control." I also call them "masters of change." There was no single, sure-fire method. Success came in many forms. Are you ready to find *your* way?

DASH

THE WAY THAT HAS WORKED for lots and lots of people is a wonderful one with the strange name of "DASH," and it has helped them eat for health. You may never have heard of it, but you are about to hear a whole lot more, because that's what this book is all about.

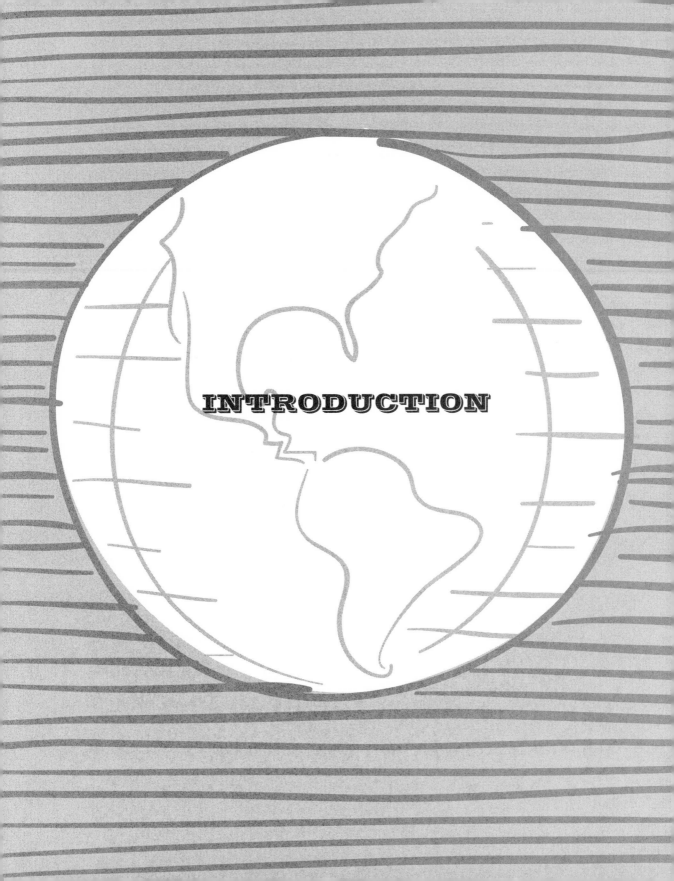

INTRODUCTION

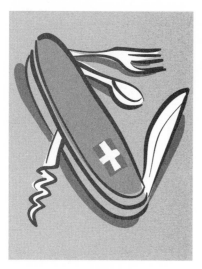

THE ALL-PURPOSE DIET

WELL, CONGRATULATIONS! You've finally found it! This is the only diet you will ever need. The all-purpose diet. This is the diet that will make you rich, famous, and healthy. Okay — healthy. ★ When you think of the word "diet," you think of "weight loss," right? In fact, we'll lay odds that's the case. You "go on a diet," which implies that at some point you're going to go off it, and most likely you're thinking "the sooner the better." You've tried diets, lots of diets, famous people's diets — maybe diets by aging actresses who used their profits to pay for the next round of cosmetic surgery (also known as "having work done"). What these diets have in common is that they claim to do everything from making you more satisfied with your life to turning you into a Greek god or goddess. The most alluring diet promise is that you'll lose weight fast, fast, fast, but, as you know all too well, "fast, fast, fast" weight loss is only temporary. Those lost pounds — and more — will be back on before you can say "hot fudge sundae," or "yo-yo," which is what you'll feel like. Frequently these diets involve pills and powders, machines and wraps, special supplements (which the diet promoters are only too happy to sell you), maybe special formulas to tell you when to eat which foods, and how to combine them for maximum efficiency (ha!). Does any of this sound familiar?

Yes, there are all sorts of short-cuts, if you believe everything you read, see, and hear. And they all have three things in common: 1) they are easy; 2) they make somebody rich (and it isn't you, you'll notice); 3) they don't work. Let's repeat that, loudly: THEY DON'T WORK!

Bouncing from diet to diet highlights one thing: body fat is complicated. If you've been unsuccessful over the long haul with a number of diets, you might want to give some extra thought to that age-old question: Why? Your body only needs a certain amount of food to keep going, so why are you eating so much more than that? If you find yourself eating virtually all the time, there's something going on besides hunger. What is it? Figure that out — you might need some help for this — and you'll clear the way for weight loss.

Losing weight is both very easy and very hard. The truth is, you eat (i.e., take in calories) and live (i.e., use calories). It's a simple formula: In order to lose weight, you have to use up more calories than you take in. It really doesn't matter what you eat, as long as you are getting rid of more than you are consuming. The more you move, the more calories you use. Yes, you even use calories when you are just sitting around, but you obviously use more if you are *moving* around, and the more vigorously you do that, the more calories you'll use. Your goal is to find a way to eat less or move more, preferably both, and watch those pounds disappear. They'll stay off, too, if you stick with the program.

There are other programs out there — you know that — and we'll mention just one of them right here: the Atkins weight-loss diet, high in fat and protein. It's also low in calories, which is why you lose weight. It's pretty limiting, pretty unbalanced, this diet, and when you limit lots of foods, you also put a lid on the calories that come from eating them. After all, how much steak and cheese can you really eat?

In a nutshell, if you are following the Atkins diet, you may find yourself dreaming of a fresh, crispy apple, a cold glass of milk, and a warm piece of bread fresh from the oven. Why? Because you aren't eating starches, fruits, vegetables, and milk. This means that you are missing out on all that these wonderful foods have to offer in the way of health — and, yes, comfort, too. It is as simple as that. Well, not quite that simple — it would be nice if you could keep that weight off. Unfortunately, as of this writing, there is no research that shows the weight stays off in the long term. No, so far there is nothing permanent about Atkins, unless you count the fact that this diet has been in and out of the public eye for the past 30 years. Do you want to give up so much for such uncertain results? Ask yourself: am I going to follow this diet for the rest of my life?

So you are finding a way. Why not find a way that offers maximum health benefits, even before you start thinking about weight loss? Health is a hot topic these days. Health segments are all over the place on both radio and television. Even TV's irreverent The Daily Show ran a segment called "You, Your Health, and You." Oddly enough, with all the talk about health, you might assume a weight loss diet would be healthy, but this is not necessarily true. Many such diets have nothing at all to do with health. As we've just seen, some remove whole food groups from your eating life.

You may be saying "So what? I'd rather be thin." Well, we are happy to report that you can lose weight and be healthy, too. An unbeatable combination.

You might as well eat in a way that will make you healthier — which does not, by the way, mean good-bye pizza, hello cardboard. It's just that you'll have pizza as an occasional treat, rather than five nights a week. Being in it for the long haul means that you will FORGET about "diet," because eating well will become second nature. Besides, it's a boring life when you have to think about food all the time. Ask anyone who has been listening to you discuss your latest diet. (Ironic, isn't it, that just when you'd love to get your mind off food, you can think of nothing else?)

In the short term, obviously, you'll have to pay some attention to all of this. But in the long term (read: the rest of your long, healthy life) you'll be able to focus on other things, like your bridge game, or winning the lottery, or patenting the "new new thing."

Here's the big news: *"Diet"* simply refers to the food you eat every day, no matter what it is. That's your diet. Ideally, the foods you choose every day are particularly good for you — like maybe fruits, vegetables, and milk, recommended by every agency in America that is responsible for your health, and your mother.

And you really do want to be healthy, right?. It sure beats not being healthy. Time spent at the doctor. Dealing with insurance. Listening to friends' advice. And on and on. When you are healthy you feel good, you look good, your clothes fit. Your friends notice that something is different, but they can't quite put their finger on it. Usually they think you got your hair cut.

How do you do all this? We like to call it "**THE HEALTHY WEIGH**." Basically this is all about making good food choices, getting yourself moving (another way of saying "exercise"), and getting yourself down to your fighting weight.

Or you may already be at your fighting weight. Fantastic! **THE HEALTHY WEIGH** is still for you, but you've gotten a jump on the weight-loss part of the deal. With that in mind (and as you've just seen), we've put in little **THE HEALTHY WEIGH** updates that will help you keep an eye on weight.

THE HEALTHY WEIGH is really about two things — the weight you take off, and the healthy way you get there. It may involve the *"14-Day Meal Plan with Meal Appeal"* that is included in this book. Or it may involve a nutrition expert putting together a specially designed meal plan. Having a plan feels good, because you have already taken a big step forward.

If you lose weight this way, IT IS WEIGHT YOU WILL NOT REGAIN. How? How? How? By doing it s-l-o-w-l-y. After all, you gained it slowly, didn't you? It took — what — five years to gain those fifty pounds? Sure, you'd like to lose it in a few months. Maybe you'd like to time travel, too, but guess what? It isn't going to happen. This is the truth (would we lie to you?), and keep in mind that knowledge is power. If you prefer Latin: *Nam et ipsa scientia potestas est.* (Francis Bacon)

While you lose weight, you gain something absolutely amazing. You decrease your risk of heart disease, high blood pressure, and diabetes. If you already have these conditions, your weight loss will

THE HEALTHY WEIGH: Secret to losing weight — eat less and move more.

THE HEALTHY WEIGH: Talk to your doctor about your weight. Get a good exam, and make sure there are no medical reasons why you are overweight.

THE HEALTHY WEIGH

The goal is to lose 10% of your weight in a year.

improve your lipids, blood pressure, and blood glucose. When you reach just 5% weight loss, you begin to see these wonderful changes. So you want to lose weight and you want to lose it in a healthy way.

This not one of those "Summer starts next week! Get into your sexy bathing suit by then!" or "I have to lose fifty pounds for my daughter's wedding in three months!" weight loss situations. Instead, you have to take a deep breath and understand reality: *You can lose, and keep off, 10% of your weight.* In a year. To repeat — you won't regain those pounds. Let your body adjust to that new weight for a few months, and then do it again — 10%. Continue this routine until you like what you see in the mirror. We know that you can lose an average of 30% and keep it off for five years. (For more on this, keep reading.) Just remember that what you see in the mirror is all about advertising and peer pressure and looking good. We can report that, on the inside too, you'll look better than ever. You won't see it, but that improved health will be there nevertheless, and your skin will look better, and your hair will be shinier, too.

You may be disappointed to discover that this is a long process. Maybe you are tempted instead to try the Telephone Pole diet, as we think of it, since it advertises on telephone poles by giving a number to call if you want to "lose 30 pounds in 30 days." But we're here to tell you that all you'll lose will be money. As a matter of fact, you'll probably also lose confidence in yourself, and will consider yourself a failure in the weight loss department. (We've seen cocktail napkins that say, "On the 30-day diet, I lost 6 days.") Fast off, fast on is the way those diets work. Too bad, but that's just the way it is.

The Telephone Pole diet won't do it, but you may like the idea of being part of a program. Okay, you can be part of a program without involving phone poles. See a dietitian, participate in hospital-based classes, or join a weight-loss club, and you'll get structure without scam. Just know that you don't necessarily have to be part of a program in order to lose weight. Anyone can do it.

Back to that 30%. There is something called the National Weight Control Registry, which tracks people who have lost weight and successfully kept it off. That's all it does. It doesn't matter how they lost the weight, whether in a program or on their own. The average weight loss maintained over a five-year period was 30%. All the "suc-

THE HEALTHY WEIGH: Weigh yourself once a week. This helps you stay on track.

cessful losers" (a phrase to love!) have in common that they made changes in the way they ate, and they exercised, too. Bottom line: they did do it, and so can you. Join the "losers"! Call 1-800-606-NWCR (6927).

THE BEST WAY TO EAT

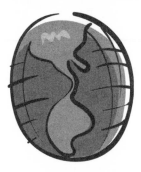

WHICH BRINGS US to the title of this book — "THE BEST DIET ON EARTH." We use the word "earth" advisedly, because, in fact, foods that come from the earth (fruits, vegetables, whole grains) are simply the best there is. Everybody says so — the ACS, AHA, ADA, AdiabA, NIH, AAP, USDA/HHS, FDA. This alphabet soup of agencies is as impressive as they come: American Cancer Society, American Heart Association, American Dietetic Association, American Diabetes Association, National Institutes of Health, American Academy of Pediatrics, US Dept of Agriculture/Health and Human Services, Food and Drug Administration.

The best diet on earth. THE BEST DIET ON EARTH! This is big stuff, important stuff, earth-shattering stuff. It just doesn't come any bigger or more important or more earth-shattering. With all the hoopla out there, with all the claims and fames, this is the one you want, because because because . . . it's the one that lowers your blood pressure, AND it reduces the risk of developing obesity, diabetes, heart disease, and certain cancers! Let's hear it for THE BEST DIET ON EARTH!

"DASH" YOUR WAY TO HEALTH

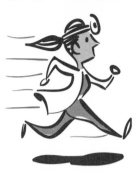

HOW DO YOU KNOW you've got the best diet on earth? You design a study, which is, after all, what the best researchers do. And that's exactly what the NIH (again — the National Institutes of Health) did. The NIH holds a very special place in our hearts, because they designed a study called "DASH," which had powerful results — so powerful, in fact, that the researchers themselves called it "the diet for all diseases." We call it THE BEST DIET ON EARTH.

"DASH" stands for "Dietary Approaches to Stop Hypertension" (also known as high blood pressure, which many people don't even know they have. That's a big deal, too, since it can cause strokes). You can see why they switched to "DASH." But a funny thing happened on the way to the nickname. We've said it before and we'll say it again: **Not only did the diet reduce blood pressure, but it turned out to be the same diet that reduces the risk of developing heart disease, obesity, osteoporosis, and certain kinds of cancer and diabetes.** If adopted nationwide, DASH would mean a 15% reduction in heart disease and a 27% decrease in stroke. See? It really is the best diet on earth.

By the way — you'll notice that there are no little numbers that send you searching through the Endnotes for further explanation. Do, though, take a look at that section in the back of this book. There you will find the studies that are the basis for all we say. There are reasons why these foods are the Best Foods on Earth — scientific reasons.

So what is DASH? Basically, it started out as a dream come true for the researchers. These happy men and woman, important researchers in the United States, looked at all the evidence for healthy eating and designed a diet they believed would most likely lower blood pressure. They had support from the NIH, the federal agency that is committed to protecting your health.

And it was certainly a dream come true for the participants, a food-preparation holiday FOR WEEKS ON END — the equivalent of an ENTIRE SUMMER — and if you were one of the participants, you never had to make a single trip to the supermarket. Your job: eat only the food provided by the research team. Not only did you get your meals every single day of the week, you also got games and parties and party favors.

Why all the attention? Because you had high blood pressure, and researchers wanted to know if food could lower it. You were being studied. Not like you were in a zoo, or anything like that. No one was looking at you, just at what you ate and how your body responded to it. Again, the whole idea was to see if the foods you ate could lower your blood pressure, thereby making you a healthier person. The answer was a resounding "yes." Quickly, too — within days, in fact. This was a huge, huge thing! **IN SOME CASES, THIS MEANT LESS MEDICATION! IN OTHER CASES, IT MEANT NO MEDICATION AT ALL!**

Are you wondering about your blood pressure? Good idea, since (we'll say it again) it can easily be high without your knowing it. Why not visit your favorite blood pressure cuff? Maybe it's at Wal-Mart. Maybe it's in a mall someplace. Certainly your doctor has one. Instead of wondering, get some information. Remember, knowledge is power. And here's some "knowledge" for you: Normal blood pressure is anything less than 120/80.

But back to the DASH study. Happily, the foods were pleasantly familiar ones, a special combination with mass appeal — that is, foods that people actually eat. Real food for real people. What exactly are these "familiar" foods? How about fruits and vegetables? How about milk? Familiar, right? People in the study liked what they ate, too. That was important.

Real foods work, and no one knows exactly why. What they do know is that food is greater than the sum of its parts, which is just another way of saying that you can't take a bunch of pills and expect the same results. It's about food, pure and simple, and what you eat is a choice you make every day, again and again. Be clear about this: Those choices affect your health, now and throughout your life.

Okay, where were we?

THE HEALTHY WEIGH: Remember — all food groups are important.

We know there really is a way to eat for health, and we know the food is familiar and good, too. What's next? Putting this into practice for yourself, so that YOU will be that "healthier person" we talk about. You already eat every day, so you might as well make some slight changes that will have a big pay-off.

There is, of course, one tiny advantage that the people in the study had. They got a lot of attention (the prepared meals, the parties, the party favors). Now comes the question — if those being studied got so much attention, who is paying attention to you? Who is making sure that you are eating well, seeing to it that you have twenty-one meals a week and the kind of little fruit snacks you took with you to elementary school?

Well, here we are. WE are paying attention to you. You are the reason we wrote this book. Maybe we can't do your food shopping, make your meals, pack your little snacks, but we're ready to help, if you are ready to let us do that.

FAST FORWARD
10 THINGS
YOU CAN DO RIGHT NOW
TO GET STARTED

① Write down everything, and we mean everything, you eat for at least three days (see pages 138-140). You have to do this *while* you're actually eating it.

② Eat three meals every day, and make them breakfast, lunch, and dinner.

③ Sit down, preferably in the kitchen or dining room, to eat your meals. Sitting in the car is not ideal.

④ While you're sitting down — plan two weeks of meals (see "14-Day Meal Plan with Meal Appeal").

⑤ Be adventurous — try a new grain or grain-like food (quinoa? wild rice?) with dinner tonight.

⑥ Think of the old "Blue Plate Special" when you plan your meal. Now update it! Fill 1/2 your plate with vegetables, 1/4 with whole grains, and 1/4 with meat, poultry, beans, whatever.

⑦ Make your plate attractive. Remember — you eat first with your eyes.

⑧ Drink a glass of milk — fat free or low fat.

⑨ Snack on fruits and vegetables.

⑩ Get moving! Walk somewhere, anywhere.

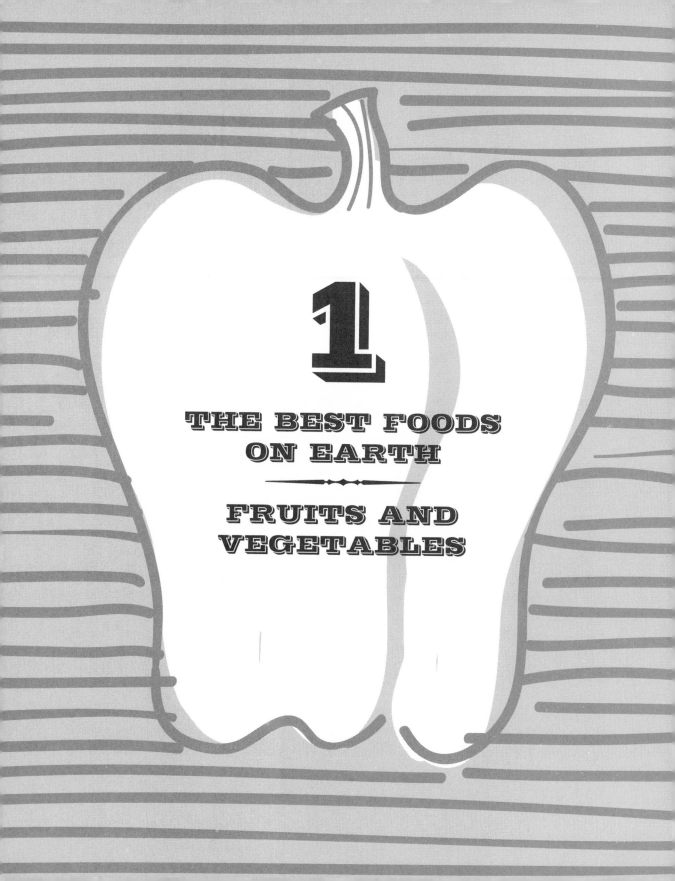

1

THE BEST FOODS ON EARTH

FRUITS AND VEGETABLES

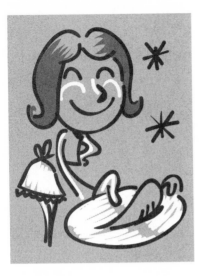

MOM KNEW BEST. She knew that fruits and vegetables are good for you (she spent a good portion of your childhood telling you to eat them), and that they are filled with vitamins and minerals. She had the right idea, even if she didn't know that, besides vitamins and minerals, they are filled with thousands of wonderful little "miracle workers" called "phytochemicals." (Pronounced FIGHT-o-chemicals. We could tell you that "phyto-" means "plant," but all we need to know is that plant foods pack a health wallop.) It turns out that these miracle workers are the stars of the new millennium: They protect the body against cancer and heart disease, prevent the formation of blood clots, and lower blood pressure. Who knows what other miracles we'll find they can perform? Yes, Mom knew best, all right. ★ To get that health wallop we referred to a minute ago, you'll want to eat a wide variety of fruits and vegetables, since different plants have different phytochemicals. Hint: an easy way to get that variety is by color, since phytochemicals are responsible for giving color to fruits and vegetables. Think of it as the "rainbow approach" to healthy eating.

FRUIT

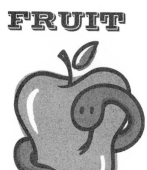

LET'S FACE IT. Fruit hasn't enjoyed the best reputation. Adam had a certain run-in with an apple, and, although we wouldn't swear to it, we suspect that incident may well have turned him off fruit entirely. His American descendants apparently still harbor an aversion to it. We know that more than half of all adults don't eat even one serving of fruit a day. That's a sobering statistic, especially when you consider that fruit is the original fast food. What could be easier access than an apple or a banana? Or grapes? Same deal, only bite size (you don't need Oreos to have bite size). Or how about oranges, conveniently packaged in nature's own shrink wrap? And there's a world of fruit out there that literally comes from all over the world, giving you a stunning variety of fruits to choose from — and endlessly in season, too. It's beautiful, it's delicious, it's available. What more could you want?

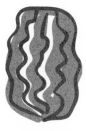

Dried, Frozen, and Canned Fruit

FRUITS CAN COME TO YOU other than fresh, and they, too, have the amazing health benefits. For some reason, people assume there is less nutrition in dried, frozen, or canned, but fruit in all these forms is healthy.

Fruits other than fresh are indeed healthy. They just last longer. Dried simply means that the water has been removed. Take away the water from grapes and we call them "raisins." Newly popular are dried blueberries and cranberries. Take away the water and we call them "blueberries" and "cranberries." Dried. You can buy "craisins," cranberries that look like raisins, as well as all sorts of mixed dried fruit tidbits.

Sun-Maid makes a number of dried fruit combinations, which can be eaten "as is" or used in recipes.

Dried and canned fruits can be as manageable and portable as fresh. We love individual serving sizes — little boxes of raisins, flip-

**THE
HEALTHY WEIGH:**
1/4 cup of dried fruit is
about right for a
serving size.

**THE
HEALTHY WEIGH:**
Drink too much juice
and you'll gain weight.
Always remember
what a serving size is:
in this case, just 3/4
cup. This is worth
remembering,
because if you drink
several times that, you
are no longer drinking
for a Healthy Weigh.
(By the way — if your
child is overweight,
take a closer look at
his or her juice-
drinking habits.)

top containers of fruit cocktail, peaches, pears, applesauce. As for frozen, portability isn't much of an issue. For obvious reasons, you're better off keeping frozen food at home and using it there. Unless, of course, you have a sore elbow and are off somewhere using it as an ice pack. (By the way — try a bag of frozen berries for this. Hard to beat.)

Fresh, frozen, or dried? Depends on your storage situation. Plenty of room in the refrigerator? Buy fresh. More room in the freezer? Stock up on frozen. If you have lots of shelf space but not much refrigerator or freezer space, and if you have a can opener, consider canned fruit. All that matters is that you eventually eat the fruit that you have put so much thought into storing.

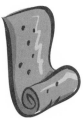

Fruit Myths

Fruit myth: If the label mentions the word "fruit," you are getting real fruit. Don't be fooled! You may not be dealing with fruit at all! Even though people are ever hopeful that foods bearing only the vaguest connection to fruit "count" as fruit (fruit-flavored yogurt, for example), the truth is, it has to look like fruit to be considered fruit. Forms of fruit do not, repeat NOT include fruit bars, fruit roll-ups, and fruit candies. Watch out for faux fruit. Go for the real thing — nature's own is always the best.

Nature's own fruit juice — "juiced fruit" — is another important form of fruit, as long as it's 100% juice. Plenty of "juices" are actually juice "drinks" (fake juice), and if you read the teeny-weeny print really, really carefully, you'll find out that you're getting only 10% juice. That's 90% something else, and the "something else" is — you guessed it — an artificially flavored, sweetened water. You are paying an awful lot for flavored water.

Real juice. It's as good as fruit because it IS fruit.

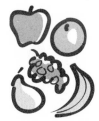

Fruit at Every Meal

IF IT'S SO IMPORTANT TO EAT FRUIT, we should discuss how much you need to eat in order to be healthy. The answer is . . . FIVE SERVINGS OF FRUIT A DAY, the magic number, the one that is associated with healthy living. And just how big are those servings? Well, a piece of fruit might be the size of a fist (not the Incredible Hulk's, however). Or a hard ball. Works for an apple, an orange, a bunch of grapes, but how about watermelon? Obviously, you'll have to cut it up to get your serving. If you can't wait to find out what that would be, see the Gory Details of Serving Sizes, page 119.

High Five! Try Five! How do you go about working it into your "eating day"? It's a simple theme: No meal without fruit. To rephrase: Fruit at every meal. And why with every meal? Because it's easy to forget, and, in fact, most Americans are forgetting to eat fruit. It's just not something they think about. But if you tie fruit-eating to meal-eating, you'll be fine. We're betting that you do eat meals, so make fruit a part of the meal, and then you'll remember to eat it.

Breakfast is the most obvious fruit meal and plays a special role in living "no meal without fruit." Juice and fruit with cereal — nothing new here. Now add fruit to take along with you and you're on your way. That's three servings already.

We're talking about fruit with each meal, and that's one down (breakfast), two to go: lunch and dinner. Do the math. If you had three pieces of fruit at breakfast, that leaves one piece of fruit at lunch and one at dinner. You'll hit that magic number (High Five! Try Five!).

While you're at it, you'll want to think beyond orange juice and bananas. Nothing wrong with them, of course. They're good choices, healthy and delicious, but you are limiting yourself unnecessarily if that's the only fruit you have. First of all, you'll wind up bored, and bored isn't great. Second, you'll deprive yourself of a whole world of tastes and health benefits that you can only get by eating a variety of fruits. That "rainbow approach" again. By the way — there are actually some fruits out there that you may never have heard of. One in particular is a real winner. A seasonal fruit, it's a cross

THE HEALTHY WEIGH: If you are trying to lose weight and are afraid you won't be able to if you eat a lot of fruit, talk to a dietitian. You just may wind up with your own personal Designer Meal Plan that will give you all the health wallop of DASH and help you lose weight, too.

between a plum and an apricot, and it's called a "pluot" in some places, an "aprium" in others. Either way, it is sweet, juicy, and altogether delicious. Then you might try exotic fruits like mango, papaya, and persimmon, for example.

Here's a shopping tip: Buy three peaches, one ripe and ready, one a little firmer, and a third that needs a few days to ripen. With a little practice you'll get good at knowing how long it will take a given peach to ripen to perfection. You can have a perfectly ripe peach daily for three days.

So there you have it — variety, variety, variety, plus a little memory aid that we call "Life With Fruit."

LIFE WITH FRUIT

Breakfast on the run?
A banana with your bun.
Grab an apple, too,
It's a simple thing to do.

Please, don't forget your juice.
(Do we sound like Dr. Seuss?)
Fruit at breakfast starts the day
It's the "High five! Try five!" way.

For lunch? A salad, please
Add pear slices (it's a breeze).
Throw in some berries now
Take a culinary bow.

With dinner — cantaloupe?
Canned peach halves? (Warm, we hope.)
Or else some cut-up fruit?
Easy living — what a hoot!

VEGETABLES

THE OTHER HALF of the fruits-and-vegetables combo is, of course, vegetables. They share the "health wallop" we talked about earlier, and, like fruits, they have those little miracle workers going to bat for them in the form of phytochemicals.

Mom was perfectly right when she told you to "Eat your vegetables!" back when they were overcooked to an unappetizing gray-green. Vegetables have come a long way.

So maybe you've listened to your mother and are already eating your vegetables, on your way to the FIVE SERVINGS OF VEGETABLES A DAY associated with healthy living. Lettuce and tomato on your sandwich. Potato and green beans (yes, potatoes are vegetables) on your dinner plate. Add a salad and you hit that magic number. High Five! Try Five! Works for fruit, works for vegetables.

You're doing fine, but we don't want you to be bored, which could well be the case if your dinner plate looks the same night after night. If it does, you are in the dreaded "veggie rut," and the way out is to eat vegetables with all sorts of different colors, shapes, textures — in other words, eat a variety of vegetables. (Why are you not surprised?) Let's take another look at that dinner plate. As a change from potatoes and green beans, why not try sweet potatoes and cooked spinach? Lima beans and carrots? Peas and mushrooms?

Here's an interesting factoid: Unlike the case with fruit, Americans do seem to be getting enough vegetables each day. That sounds pretty good, doesn't it? Well, it sounds more hopeful than it is. Things like french fries count as vegetables (we've just seen that potatoes are vegetables, "starchy" vegetables, actually), and we all know that french fries are very popular. We know for a fact that Americans are eating lots and lots of french fries. The vegetables they are not getting are the dark green ones.

We've already said that both fruits and vegetables are loaded with those little miracle workers known as "phytochemicals," and that these are protective in many ways. If you eat lots of different vegeta-

THE HEALTHY WEIGH, 1827 VERSION: It's always been easy to overcook vegetables. "If vegetables are a minute or two too long over the fire, they lose their beauty and flavor." Robert Roberts, "The House Servant's Directory," 1827

THE HEALTHY WEIGH, 1828 VERSION: See how long green vegetables have been an important part of a beautiful plate? "Ham should always be accompanied by a green vegetable such as asparagus, beans, spinach, broccoli." Directions for Cookery. Published in Philadelphia by Eliza Leslie in 1828.

**THE
HEALTHY WEIGH:**
If weight loss is your
issue, you have a
pleasant choice to
make: Nonstarchy
vegetables, of which
you can eat pretty
much unlimited
quantities, provided
they are not fried,
smothered in sauce,
etc.; you know the drill.
Or starchy vegetables
which can put the
weight on if you eat a
lot of them. Your
choice. Which is which,
you are wondering?
Examples of
nonstarchy are
broccoli, carrots, and
cauliflower. Examples
of starchy are peas,
corn, and potatoes.
Our recommendation
is to choose some of
each, with the above
information firmly in
mind. Still in doubt?
Get a little help with
your own Designer
Meal Plan that will give
you all the health
wallop of vegetables,
both starchy and
nonstarchy, and will
help you lose weight,
too.

bles, you'll reap the benefits of as many phytochemicals as possible.

Certainly the good news is that there are more vegetables to choose from. What's also new is that there are more shortcuts. Here's to the manufacturers who have done all the work, or almost all of it, so that you can move forward with the business of cooking (if necessary) and eating (definitely necessary). You'll find tiny little carrots, peeled and washed; shredded cabbage; cute little pieces of broccoli, ditto cauliflower; sliced mushrooms, bite-size grape tomatoes, and more.

Salad Alley

SO NOW THAT YOU HAVE these nice vegetables all cut up and ready for you, a true shortcut is to make a salad. You get lots of vegetables at once, and you eliminate the cooking. (The shortest cut of all salad-wise is to buy your salad at a supermarket salad bar, but that gets pretty expensive if you're making salad for several people.)

There is a price to pay for this convenience. Prepackaged food is more expensive, but, fortunately, you have a range of other options as you collect your salad fixings. Don't let money be your excuse to avoid eating salad. You might choose instead to buy vegetables in bulk (Hint: you'll be pleasantly surprised at the prices at produce markets), and cut them up yourself.

Now all you have to add is lettuce. Maybe you'll go for the see-through package of pre-washed lettuce, winner of the coveted Convenience Award for tool-free preparation. It is literally the leader of the pack. Or maybe you'd rather wash and spin your own lettuce with a salad spinner, both a wildly useful tool and a boon to people who used to let their lettuce dry on towels spread all over the kitchen — and dining room too — when company was coming. This "homespun" lettuce can be stored for several days in the refrigerator if bagged in plastic with some paper towels to absorb extra moisture. It will be all ready to go when it's time to make your salad.

We like a combination approach. We add pre-washed/packaged salad fixings to our homespun salad, thereby "stretching" the more expensive stuff.

Let's face it — there are times when no amount of help in the way of packaged salad is enough to convince us to make a salad, let alone dinner. That doesn't mean we don't want to eat a salad, just that we don't want to be the ones to make it. Those are the times when we go to a restaurant, which might be just a fast-food place with a good salad bar. This allows us to skip preparation entirely and go directly to eating the salad.

Bottom line: If you think "limp lettuce" when you think of salad, think again. Do whatever you have to do in order to eat salad every day. It's increasingly popular. Try adding a sliced apple or a hefty amount of cut-up melon. Even a melon that isn't as sweet as you'd hoped it would be does very well when tossed in a salad, where it gets coated with a good dressing. Throw in some nuts (walnuts? almonds? what do you like?) and seeds (sunflower? pumpkin?). They add a great taste and a wonderful crunch.

Don't be surprised if at some point the ever-popular National Secretaries Week, well known for the time when secretaries are taken out for lunch, is followed by Salad Appreciation Day, with greeting cards suggesting you "Take A Salad To Lunch." Strange but true, salads build relationships and can even be aphrodisiacs. We were standing in line at a buffet dinner and overheard someone exclaim, "I want to marry the person who made that salad!"

By the way — we believe that salad dressing is a good place to use healthy oils (olive, canola, nut oils).

Are you an iceberg fan? You have only to remember the Titanic to know that icebergs don't have what you'd call an enviable reputation. They don't pack much of a health wallop, either, being so pale and all. Try a darker leaf lettuce. That's where the good stuff is.

SALAD DAYS

When we're not in such a hurry
And our minds are free from worry,
Then we buy a head or two
(Any lettuces will do).
Next, we get the salad spinner
'Cause it's almost time for dinner,
Spin those leaves until they're dry —
Spinners work! Give one a try!
But if we're really busy
And in something of a tizzy
And our spirits sort of sag,
We buy lettuce in a bag.
It's pre-washed, and not by us,
Which eliminates the fuss.
But sometimes, though it's rare,
Even that is hard to bear.
So if we're feeling weary
And the kitchen's looking dreary
And we need a special treat —
Well, then we go out to eat.
We make sure to order salad
'Cause we're looking pretty pallid.
Here's the last thing we will say:
Eat your SALAD every day!

"Cauliflower is
nothing but a
cabbage with a
college education."
— Mark Twain

Vegetables Every Day

SOME PEOPLE LIKE VEGETABLES only if they are fried or covered with a cream or cheese sauce, at which point they are vegetables in disguise. That is, they don't look like the original, they don't taste like the original, but most important, they don't pack the complete health wallop of the original. Potatoes, for example, are frequently disguised — deep fried (think "french fries" and potato chips), or drowned in a rich sauce (think "scalloped"). The award for Best Disguise goes to batter-dipped, deep fried vegetables. Vegetables, which started life as low-fat foods, suddenly aren't. They're not low in fat, and they sure aren't low in calories. They, like all vegetables in disguise, move into the realm of "Special Occasion Vegetables," which has less to do with the vegetables themselves than with their preparation.

So you fry only on special occasions. That leaves a lot of days for Everyday Vegetables, which can be cooked in any number of ways. Need some ideas? Read on.

VEGGIES EVERY WAY

You can roast 'em
You can toast 'em
You can tell your friends and boast 'em.
You can steam 'em
While you're dreamin',
You can simmer
(And get slimmer)
You can grill
And get your fill.
You can sauté, you can bubble,
'Cause it isn't any trouble,
You can cook 'em any way.
Just eat your veggies EVERY DAY!

Our next-to-last line could have been "You can cook 'em any way — except frying," but then it wouldn't have rhymed.

THE HEALTHY WEIGH:
If you fry or cover your vegetables with a buttery or cheesy sauce, you are not eating the healthy way.

IN A NUTSHELL:
Start today! Choose fruits and vegetables with an eye toward color. Lots of colors = lots of miracle workers in your corner.

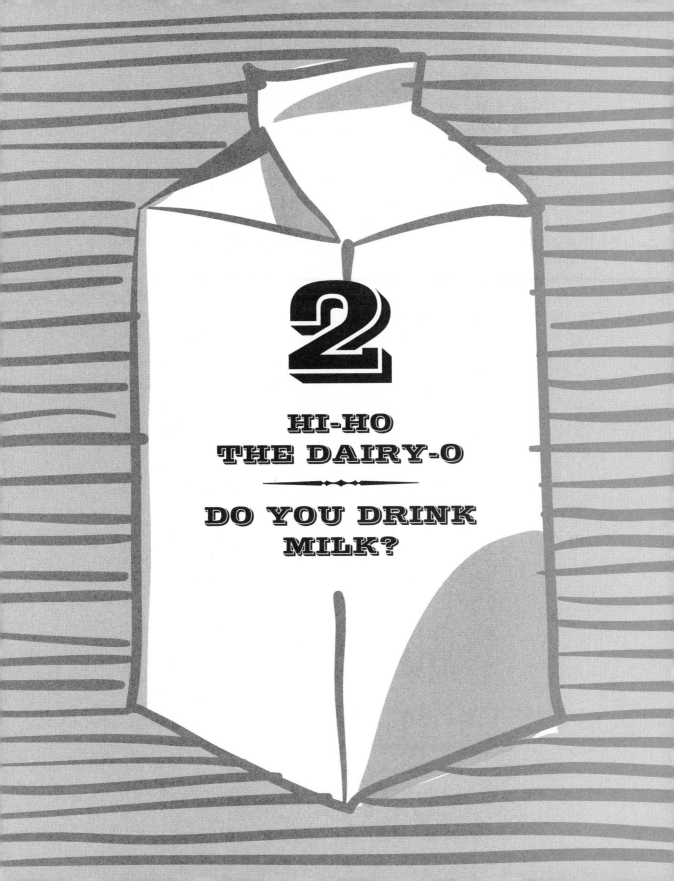

2

HI-HO
THE DAIRY-O

DO YOU DRINK
MILK?

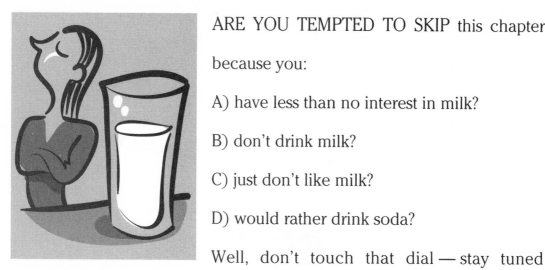

ARE YOU TEMPTED TO SKIP this chapter because you:

A) have less than no interest in milk?

B) don't drink milk?

C) just don't like milk?

D) would rather drink soda?

Well, don't touch that dial — stay tuned to…MILK. You already know it's good for bones, and maybe you take a calcium pill for just that reason, which is fine. But there's more to milk than calcium, and we're just finding out how much more. Milk packs another powerful health wallop, and there are wonderful mysteries unraveling about its protective properties — protecting the heart, protecting from breast cancer, protecting young adults from eventually developing adult onset diabetes. Apparently there is more to come. What we already know is that two to three cups of milk a day, combined with fruits and vegetables, lowers blood pressure without medication! (To clarify: Some people do not need any medication at all, and others need it, but perhaps less of it.) ★ What if you've never liked milk? Give yourself a few weeks to learn to like it. Because you are fully committed to taking care of yourself, chances are that, in time, you'll figure out a way to get milk into your day. Fortunately, tastes change. Start slowly and give it a try. You might surprise yourself. Think of drinking milk as putting on shining armor, protecting you all your life, not just when you were a kid. No, milk isn't just for kids anymore, but most adults don't realize that, and they are shortchanging themselves by not drinking it. Consider that half of women, two thirds of men, and almost all teenage girls are choosing not to have the protective armor of milk.

Obviously, you have lots of company if you are not a milk-drinker, but the benefits of drinking milk are such that you might want to reconsider your position.

Drink milk. You'll be glad you do.

LEAVE THE FAT BEHIND

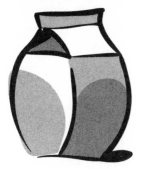

SO NOW YOU'RE DRINKING MILK. Many happy returns! Just be aware that there is something in there that you don't want, and that something is fat, saturated fat. It enjoys a particularly bad reputation, associated as it is with heart disease. As good as milk is for you, the fat is a downside. Do you really want mixed messages in your milk? There's a lot of fat in whole milk, less in reduced fat, even less in low fat, and none in fat free (hence the name). Obviously, you'll want to go with low fat or fat free. If you are used to drinking whole milk, switch first to reduced fat, then to low fat, and then to fat free. We know, we know. Compared to whole milk, low fat and fat free taste watery. But persevere. Soon enough these milks will taste light and fresh to you, and the higher fat milks will seem too heavy. If the lower fat milks continue to strike you as too thin, check out the thicker skim milks now on the market. The label may say "non-fat milk with the rich taste of 2%." More protein and calcium make these milks "richer." The carton will tell you to shake first. That's the milk, not you.

MILK PROBLEMS

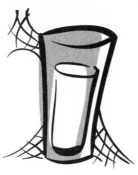

YOU MAY THINK that you can't drink milk because it doesn't agree with you. In fact, if you haven't been drinking milk for a long time, you may have lost your ability to process it. But it's like riding a bike. Get back on and you'll be amazed at how quickly the ability returns. Start slowly, and soon you'll be able to drink an 8-ounce glass of milk with no problem. Then, later in the day, have another glass. You're aiming for two to three glasses a day, and you're there already. Sometimes things work out.

Some people, however, simply cannot tolerate milk. Is this you? Do you have trouble digesting a part of the milk called "lactose"? Relief is on the way, and you don't have to give up milk, either. You can buy a specially designed milk called "Lactaid" at the grocery store. When this milk is not available (at work? out to dinner?), you can take a Lactaid caplet or chew a tablet when you drink a glass of ordinary milk. Lactaid-on-the-go.

"MILK"

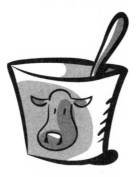

WHY THE QUOTATION MARKS? Well, the two to three cups of milk you drink can take other forms. That is, it doesn't have to be milk, it can come from milk. Then it's called "dairy." Think yogurt. Like grape-juice that ferments and becomes wine, milk ferments and becomes yogurt, retaining the protective properties of milk, and then some. An 8-ounce container of yogurt pretty much equals a cup of milk. As far as fat goes — same deal as milk, with full fat, low-fat and fat-free versions available. Choose wisely.

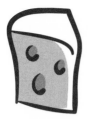

Hi-Ho the Dairy-O, the Cheese Stands Alone

GOOD NEWS DEPARTMENT: Milk can take the form of cheese! One-and-a-half ounces of cheese, like 8 ounces of yogurt, equals about one cup of milk. Like milk, cheese is an excellent source of calcium and protein, but it is also an excellent source of fat, so if you are getting your calcium and protein from cheese, you'll have to go with low fat or fat free. Now, because we are a nation of cheese-lovers-who-are-trying-to-lower-their-fat-intake, cheese manufacturers are proud to offer these low-fat and fat-free cheeses. You will, however, have to change your expectation of cheese when you try these products.

Fat-free cheese melts a little differently, which you may or may not like. Experiment with the melt-factor of different cheeses and different brands. Try Cabot, Alpine Lace, Kraft. Definitely try it (unmelted!) in your salad, where it will add a nice flavor and texture, and make the salad more of a meal. You may even enjoy the process of cutting it up, since it has such an interesting feel. By the way, if you drop a piece on the floor, you'll notice it bounces.

Or you can use low-fat cheeses (no more than 3 grams of fat per ounce), which have the advantage of better "melt-ability," but the disadvantage that the fat adds up quickly if you eat a lot. You could also stay with old-fashioned cheese, the kind mother used to buy, and just use less of it. This is fine if you can convince yourself that 1/4 cup of grated cheese sprinkled over an entire casserole is enough. But if you can already picture yourself scraping off the entire cheese layer and putting it on your own plate, you'd do well to consider eliminating cheese from your day-to-day diet. This doesn't mean that you'll never have any more cheese. It simply means that cheese moves away from the everyday and into the realm of "occasional treat."

THE HEALTHY WEIGH: If you're a cheese lover, here's a tip: More is not better. You may be hoping that cheese, like fruits and vegetables, is in the "High five! Try five!" camp. Sorry, but it's not. By the way, always make sure the small amounts of cheese you do eat are low fat or fat free. Ditto milk.

MILK IMPOSTERS

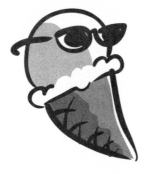

A WORD OF CAUTION. There are products out there that sound like dairy, look like dairy, and turn up in the dairy or freezer section of the grocery store. However, they don't have what it takes to walk hand-in-hand with milk, because they are missing key players: calcium and protein. In other words, you think you are in the presence of a milk product but you're not. The most common of these imposters are old-fashioned cream cheese, sour cream, cottage cheese (yes, cottage cheese can be an imposter!), ice cream, and frozen yogurt. Unfortunately, you can't count them as milk.

Manufacturers work hard to develop enticing imposters. Special mention must be made of yogurt-covered raisins and berries. Although it sounds like you're getting milk with your dried fruit, what you're really getting is candy. Too bad. It seemed like such a good idea.

THE HEALTHY WEIGH:

Use the Nutrition Facts to see if your low-fat dairy is a milk or an imposter. If a serving (8 ounces) is about 90 calories, 8 grams of protein and 25% or more of calcium, you have a real, honest-to-goodness milk.

DAIRY EVERY DAY

YOU KNOW WHAT TO DO. Have some cereal with your milk. Have some dinner with your milk. Put milk in a wine glass and feel like royalty. And you won't have a headache the next day, either. Make a velvet drink with fruit and milk or yogurt (see recipe for FAST AND FRUITY BREAKFAST on page 198). Yummy yum yum. Take a container of yogurt to work. Snack with milk, and pair it with a piece of fruit, maybe a banana.

But if you're still not sure what to do, try this on for size:

HI-HO, THE DAIRY-O
(TUNE: "THE FARMER IN THE DELL")

Fit milk into your day,
At work or when you play,
Hi-Ho, the Dairy-o
Fit milk into your day.

Drink two cups, even three,
Milk's not just for your tea,
Hi-Ho, the Dairy-o
Drink two cups, even three.

Try drinking milk with meals,
And see if it appeals,
Hi-Ho, the Dairy-o
Try drinking milk with meals.

Oh, have some dairy, please,
Have yogurt, have some cheese,
Hi-Ho, the Dairy-o
Oh, have some dairy, please.

Buy dairy low in fat,
Please, please remember that,
Hi-Ho, the Dairy-o
Buy dairy low in fat.

IN A NUTSHELL:
Start today! Practice drinking m-i-l-k MILK.

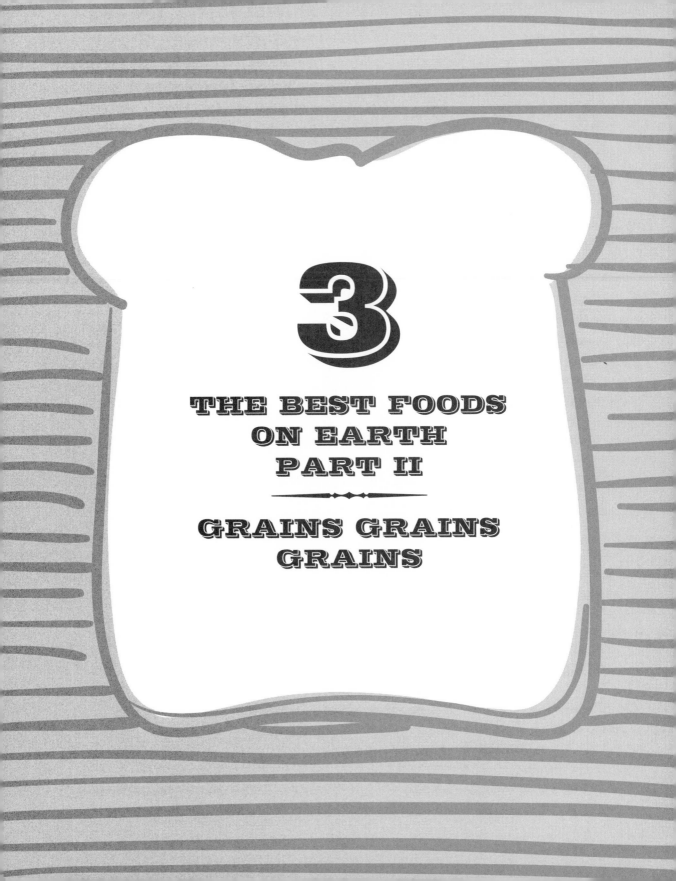

3

THE BEST FOODS ON EARTH PART II

GRAINS GRAINS GRAINS

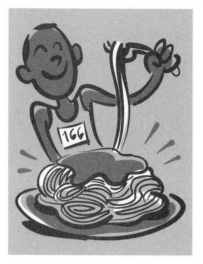

GRAINS ARE JUST PLAIN GOOD FOR YOU. There's no other way to say it. Good for you good for you good for you. The fact that grains are healthy doesn't come as any news. People have known for a long time that grains give you energy (example: eating lots of pasta before a marathon; better if you're running it, not watching on television). If you are going for health, you're going with grains. Grains and health, hand in hand. No doubt you already know this, and so we have a question: Do you eat grains? Really, do you? Of course you do. You're eating grains all the time, because they "crop" up (ha ha) all over the place. By far the most common grain in the American diet is wheat, and you find it in bagels, English muffins, bread sticks, tortillas, pita, pretzels, crackers, waffles, pancakes, pasta. ★ So the answer to the question "Do you eat grains?" is a loud "yes." A follow-up question, please: Do you eat *whole* grains? If you are anything like most Americans, the answer is, "Probably not enough." ★ Whole grains are where you want to be. For awhile everybody was talking about fiber in grain (remember oat bran?), but the rest of the grain was pretty much lost in the rush. Now we know that whole grain (clearly an endless source of fascination to somebody) has a lot more to it than energy and fiber. Whole grains — which are, like fruits and vegetables, plants, after all — have those phytochemical/miracle workers going for them. Why not put them to use for you? They are standing at attention, ready to be pressed into service.

THE "WHOLE" STORY: Common Whole Grains

OKAY, SO IT'S WHOLE GRAINS that give you the most bang for the buck. Essentially they are grains that haven't been tampered with, which means you're eating the whole thing. Simple. You've heard of "whole wheat," and that's what it is — the whole grain. Obviously if you eat the whole grain, you're going to be getting as many of those little miracle workers as possible in your corner. Try whole wheat pasta and whole wheat couscous. And why not eat other whole grains, too? Like corn, oats, barley, rice (both brown and wild), and rye, all common whole grains.

What makes whole grain so special? Scientist have studied lots of people for long periods of time and found that *whole grain reduces the risk of heart disease, cancer, and stroke, and offers protection from the kind of diabetes that develops in adulthood.* Listen up, because this is a BIG DEAL!

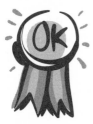

Genuine Whole Grains

IF YOU ARE WITHIN REACH of a loaf of multi-grain bread, take a look at the ingredients. By the way, we really hope you *are* within reach of a loaf of *genuine* multi-grain bread, which would encourage us a lot. Then we'd know you're already on the way. Why "genuine"? Your bread just might be an imposter. It may contain just a trace of whole grain, and it may be colored to look like whole grain. So how do you know it's genuine? Have you looked at

THE HEALTHY WEIGH: Here's a question — Can you lose weight eating grains? Answer — yes, with the right serving size. A serving of cooked grain is about the size of an ice cream scoop. Just remember to fill the scoop with a cooked grain, not ice cream.

THE HEALTHY WEIGH:

Choose whole grains.

Back in the 1800's, people were concerned about white bread. Presbyterian clergyman Sylvester Graham attacked it, saying "white bread is injurious to your health." Harriet Beecher Stowe wasn't too fond of white bread either. She and her older sister, Catherine, described store-bought bread as being "light indeed, so light that it seems to have neither weight not substance, but with no more sweetness or taste than so much cotton wool." "The American Woman's Home," 1869

your label lately? You want it to say "WHOLE." Not all breads are created equal; whole grain bread is more equal than others.

You'll find a list that looks something like this: "whole wheat, wheat, oats, rye, barley, rice, buckwheat, bulgur, and millet."

If you are really paying attention, you'll have noticed that the list of grains begins with "whole wheat" and "wheat." Maybe you thought it was a misprint, but no, whole wheat and wheat are not the same. You want to make sure that *whole* wheat, or some other *whole* grain, is the first ingredient listed. You'll also see the word "WHOLE" on the package.

Manufacturers are proud that their product meets government standards and can be labeled "whole" (read "healthy"), a badge of honor. Another badge of honor is the whole grain health claim on the package. In order for the food to make this claim, it must contain all portions of the grain kernel, contain 51% whole grain per serving, and of course be low in fat, saturated fat, and cholesterol. This is the exact wording of the health claim you will see: *"Diets rich in whole grain foods and other plant foods and low in total fat, saturated fat, and cholesterol, may reduce the risk of heart disease and some cancers."*

YOU AND YOUR BREAD

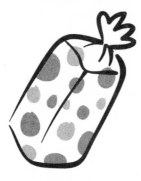

WHAT'S YOUR BREAD HISTORY? Are you still buying your childhood bread? The soft stuff that some people think of as "raw," others think of as "the bread that doesn't spoil," and still others think of as "the bread you can play with"? Studies show that some people object to the color of grain bread (that is, it's not white), but fear not. We are starting to see "white whole wheat" bread in the supermarket. Seriously. We're not kidding. White. Whole. Wheat.

Whatever bread you buy, maybe you mindlessly buy the same thing again and again, week in and week out. Are you a squeezer, checking for softness? Do you look at the date? The price? That's fine if you do any — or all — of these, but remember, now you'll be adding one more item to your checklist: Make sure that whole wheat, or some other whole grain, is the first ingredient listed. Of course if there's that shortcut — the word "WHOLE" on the package — you won't even have to check the ingredient list.

Develop a new bread history. Be adventurous. Expand your search to include bread made from rye or oats, for example. While you're at it, look for whole grain rolls (your local coffee shop may have one you particularly like), and maybe hamburger buns, too, admittedly not easy to find. Your search, if successful, will have been worth it. Your new bread history might also include thin, round, flat breads such as whole grain pita and tortillas. If your only bread is the stuff that surrounds a fast-food hamburger, you can be sure you have not begun to scale the heights of grain excellence.

FEAR OF BREAD

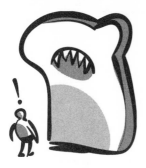

IT MAY BE THAT YOU HAVE BREAD-PHOBIA, because you've heard that it causes weight gain. Bread won't cause weight gain. Whole loaves, on the other hand, will, as will whole boxes or bags (if that is your serving size) of other bread-related products like bagels, English muffins, bread sticks, tortillas, pita, pretzels, and crackers. Obviously, *whole grain* bread won't cause weight gain, either, and if you eat whole grain breads, you'll find them pretty satisfying, so you probably won't be tempted to overdo the serving size.

Don't worry about eating bread. It's a good thing to do.

THE
HEALTHY WEIGH:
You can lose weight even if you are eating bread, whole grain or any other. If there's butter and cream cheese on it, that's another story. Then there's the issue of Own Personal Serving Size. Does your "1 serving" equal "1 loaf"? There's your problem.

THE
HEALTHY WEIGH:
Eating muffins, even when they say "whole" grain, can keep you from losing weight. One big muffin has somewhere in the neighborhood of 500 calories. One week is somewhere in the neighborhood of seven days, so if you have one of those headlight-size snacks every morning, that would be 3500 calories a week. And guess what? It happens that 3500 calories equals one pound. Your weight loss diet might well turn into a weight GAIN diet, to the tune of a pound a week.

BEYOND WHEAT

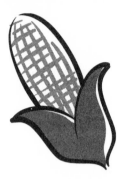

BESIDES WHOLE WHEAT there are other whole grains, everyday grains, some more familiar than others, and we've introduced them already — corn, oats, barley, rice (both brown and wild), and rye. Then there's buckwheat and bulgar, maybe less familiar. There are other grains or grain-like foods that are close to being unknown, and we'll introduce just one. Quinoa (pronounced "KEEN-wa," and winner of the award for most surprising pronunciation) is lovely and pearly and somewhat barley-like. It is tiny and delicate, with a pretty little ring in the middle. Try the quinoa recipe in the back of this book (Quinoa Wow, page 167). Think variety, and remember the little miracle workers.

THE BREAKFAST CONNECTION

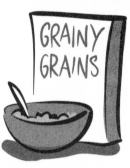

BREAKFAST IS THE KEY to eating whole grains. It's possible to get a wide variety of whole grains by eating cold cereal, so you won't have to do any cooking. (You'll get some milk in there, too — low fat or fat free, remember — and while you're at it, make sure to slurp up that milk when you've finished the cereal.) Cereals have been around for a long time and have always been associated with healthy living. Walk down the cereal aisle and you'll see some whole grain cereals that you didn't even know existed — Kashi GoLean, for instance. It has seven whole grains. Take the cereal challenge: How many whole grains does your cereal have?

Have some oats for breakfast, in the form of oatmeal. A very special grain, it protects your heart as well as manages diabetes, and it can also give you a wonderful feeling of being satisfied.

THE HEALTHY WEIGH: For achievement, intelligence, energy, weight loss, and good health, start your day with breakfast.

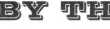
BY THE WAY...

YOU DON'T HAVE TO GIVE A THOUGHT to the fat content in whole grains because one of the nice things about them is that they are naturally low in fat. Popcorn, for example, is a whole grain that makes a great snack — provided you get a low-fat version out of your microwave, not a high-fat version at the movie theatre. All you need to know is that butter (or oil) is fat, and if that has been added, fat has been added. There are no labels on movie theatre popcorn, but the grease on your hands tells you all you need to know.

In the supermarket, of course, you can just glance at the food label. (If you can get the necessary information with a "glance," hats off to you.) For handy label-reading information, see "Labels: Keeping Track Of Fat In Packaged Foods," page 70.

If you have a sweet tooth, you probably aren't getting enough whole grains. When hunger strikes, if sweets are in the running, they will win, hands down. Grains — and you — will be the unfortunate loser.

You have some history to examine so that you'll be better equipped to plan for the future. How do you make yourself healthy? By choosing healthy whole grains over candy, cake, and cookies.

MEASURING UP

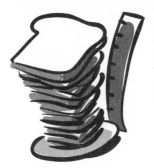

NOW THAT YOU KNOW you'll be eating grains, the only question is how much, and the answer is at least six servings a day. What is considered a serving? Good question!

☞ For breads, it's a slice
☞ For cold cereals, it's a cup
☞ For pasta and rice, it's half a cup

Can't find your measuring cup? No problem, you've got one with you.

THE HEALTHY WEIGH: Whole grains make you feel full, which is good, because then you'll eat less. Voilà — weight loss.

Cup both hands together and that's about a cup. One hand — half a cup. Easy. But you might want to look for that measuring cup, or you'll spend an awful lot of time washing your hands.

PATRIOTIC DUTY

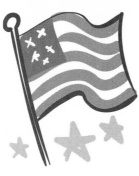

BELIEVE IT OR NOT, there is a government sponsored "Healthy People 2010" objective, and getting Americans to eat more grains is one of the goals. In other words, it is your duty as an American citizen to eat more whole grains by the year 2010. Your country needs you! You might as well get started, and not leave it to the last minute (2009) like you used to do when you had a term paper due.

Okay, you're ready to serve your country, but what does that mean? How much of this stuff do you have to eat to be considered a patriot? You just saw that you need six serving of grains every day, but your patriotism involves making sure half of those servings are whole grains (that's three, for the non-mathematically-inclined). *THREE IS THE KEY*. Have a cup of whole grain cereal for breakfast (look for the word "whole" on the box), a sandwich made from whole wheat bread for lunch, and some brown rice for dinner. If brown rice doesn't appeal, have a multi-grain roll instead — or double up at breakfast, and have a slice of whole grain toast with your cereal.

**THE
HEALTHY WEIGH:**

Make those three servings of whole grains the right serving size for a healthy weight:

> **Bread = 1 slice**
> **Cereal = 1 cup**
> **Pasta + rice = 1/2 cup**

IN A NUTSHELL:
Start today! Buy a loaf WHOLE GRAIN bread, and have a slice.

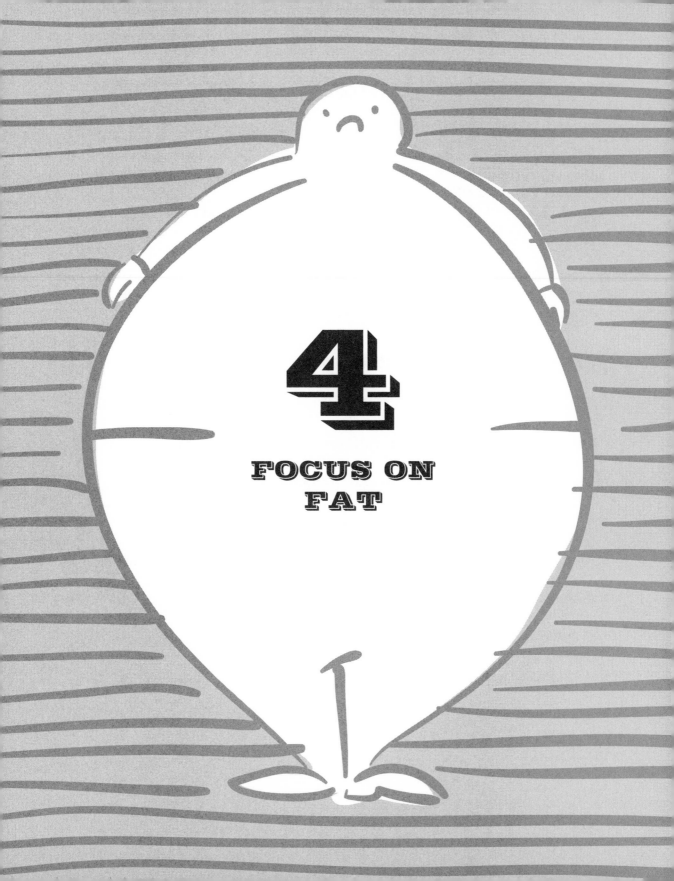

4

FOCUS ON
FAT

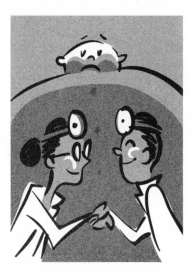

TEN YEARS AGO we wrote a book about eating low fat, because it was the healthy way to eat — and it still is. No, things haven't changed on that front. How refreshing! It's nothing short of confusing and frustrating when conflicting health information comes your way, but that is not the case here.

SAT FAT — THE KILLER FAT

LET'S START WITH SATURATED FAT, the worst of the dietary offenders, the fat most closely associated with heart disease. A "killer fat," you might say. Doesn't sound all that great, does it? It lurks menacingly in meats, poultry, and all other foods that come from animals. You might want to take another look at how much you eat in a given day, since cutting down on the amount of meat and poultry you eat will, at the same time, reduce the amount of saturated fat you consume. *It all comes down to the fact that cutting down on your serving size is the most important of all dietary changes.* Yet people resist doing this, continuing to eat large amounts of meat and poultry every day.

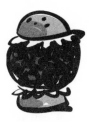

High Protein, High Sat Fat

IT'S EASY ENOUGH to see why people have trouble cutting down on the size of meat servings. Meat and poultry have customarily occupied a privileged place on the dinner plate, with the rest of the meal built around it. The time-honored question "What's for dinner?" is not looking for "baked potato," or any other side dish, as the answer. We are a nation of meat-eaters, big meat-eaters. (Too big, as a matter of fact, but the fattening-up of the population at large is another story.)

One more reason people continue to eat a lot of meat and poultry is that they know that meat is high in protein, a good thing for the body, so they assume that more is better. Books have been written advocating high protein diets, and lots of people have been sold on the idea. Keep in mind that there's a lot of saturated fat associated with all that protein, and we know its reputation. Not good. And sad but true, there's little or no place in high protein diets for the best food on earth: fruits, vegetables, milk, and whole grains. Most importantly, large amounts of protein are not health protective in any way.

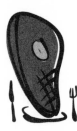

Less Is More

LET'S GET BACK to how much meat you eat, and the assumption that "more is better." Remember, meat is where the sat fat is. If you've ever been to a steak house, you've been introduced to outlandish portions, 16-ounce steaks that have to be served on incredibly large plates — let's face it, platters. Shouldn't you be able to fit your food onto a normal-size dinner plate? If you find yourself eating from serving platters, you might want to rethink portion size.

MEAT-LOVIN' STELLA
There once was a woman named Stella,
Whose steak made a lovely umbrella.
Kept her dry when it rained,
But people complained
When she took it aboard the Acela.

THE HEALTHY WEIGH: High protein diets are not the healthy way.

A 16-ounce steak may be more outlandish than you realize. The recommended serving size for meat and poultry is — you'd better be lying down for this — 3 ounces, something like a deck of playing cards. Here's a tip: If you cook your own meat, you may have heard that you should "allow for shrinkage," which is to say that the meat weighs more before it's cooked than after. That's true, but you can't buy a slab of meat the size of a Kleenex box and expect the cooked weight to be appropriate for a single serving. To put it in perspective, if you buy a pound of lean ground beef, by the time you allow for shrinkage during cooking (25 percent), that pound of beef will make four 3-ounce hamburgers. Note that this is just a rule of thumb. Move away from gigantic and toward sensible. You don't have to get crazy on the subject.

IRVING THE CAREFUL

There once was a fellow named Irving,
Three ounces of meat was his serving.
He never ate more —
But when he kept score —
Folks found it completely unnerving.

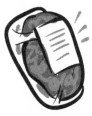

Moving Away From Sat Fat

YOU'RE EATING MEAT, but what to buy? You want lean, not fatty, so look for the words "Extra Lean" or "Lean" on the package. Extra Lean has half the fat and saturated fat of Lean. If those words are on the label, you'll know that the meat is acceptable as long as you eat only 3 ounces. If you don't see the words "Extra Lean" or "Lean" on the package, look at the Nutrition Facts label.

And what if there are no Nutrition Facts on the package, which may well be the case? You'll have to ask the butcher. Annoying, isn't it? For some reason, the USDA (United States Department of Agriculture), responsible for the labeling of meats, has dragged its heels in demanding labels from manufacturers. Consumers deserve accurate, easy-access information. They shouldn't have to play "Ask the Butcher."

Here's a **lean meat**-selecting shortcut: Meats that have the words "loin" or "round" associated with them ("pork loin," "tenderloin," "top round," "bottom round," and so on) are lean. Just remember to pick "loin" and "round" and you'll be okay. While you're at it: Before cooking the meat, use a sharp knife or scissors to trim off extra fat. Then you'll have a cut of meat that's as lean as lean can be.

If you buy your meats at a meat market that specializes in the tastiest cuts in town, you may be buying a "prime" cut of meat, which it will say on the label or be advertised as such in the store. Prime cuts are expensive and marbled with fat, the very reason they're juicier — and also fattier. Too bad that's saturated fat they're marbled with.

It should come as no surprise that the fattier meats taste good. Why else is fat so popular? It tastes great! If it didn't, there would be no discussion.

MEET MEAT
The top of the line is called "prime";
Its taste is completely sublime.
The trouble is that
It's loaded with fat,
Though pleasantly easy to rhyme.

The leanest is "loin," also "round."
Of course, they are sold by the pound.
They're the ones we prefer –
For him and for her –
The healthiest cuts we have found.

Ground beef is in a different category altogether. Don't ask us why this should be, but the FDA rules of "Lean" and "Extra Lean" do not apply to ground beef. Instead, the term "percent lean" rears its ugly head, as big letters on the package announce that the meat is "94% lean," for example, which sounds pretty good, but isn't. Worst of all, and a real insult to consumers, is the fact that there is no consistency from one store to another as to how much fat there really is in that 94% lean. *Go for the highest percentage*, which does not,

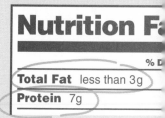

unfortunately, guarantee truly lean ground beef (less than 10 grams of fat for 3 ounces). A better option is to have the butcher grind loin or round that you can take home with confidence and know you have indeed bought truly lean ground beef.

Lunch meats, like ground beef, often use percentages — say, "97% fat free." Sounds all right, but this is very, very misleading, making you think the product is low in fat even though it isn't. Labels for all other foods must tell you how much fat is in the food. Lunch meats alone get to tell you how much fat is NOT in the food.

Let's look at what they mean by "% fat free." The percentage is by weight, which is boosted if water is added during processing. If you were able to take out the water from a lunch meat that calls itself "97% fat free" and then weigh it, you'd see that the lunch meat may be as much as 50% fat, not 97% fat free at all. On the other hand, you know you are choosing better lunch meats when they say *"fat free"* or *"low fat"* on the package.

The real point is this: Why buy lunch meats in the first place? Sliced beef (eye of round), ham, or turkey are genuine lunch meats. Those that masquerade as lunch meats share only the vaguest family history with cows and pigs and chickens, which makes you wonder why they are called "meats" in the first place. They come packaged in perfect squares and circles and have names like "bologna" and "olive loaf." When was the last time you took a child to a petting zoo to see an olive loaf? Don't buy lunch meats and assume you are buying meat. You're paying a lot of money for water and fat.

Ground meat and lunch meats are examples of absurd labeling that are unnecessarily confusing to consumers. Buyer beware.

THE HEALTHY WEIGH:

Chicken wings are better for chickens than for people. Don't eat them.

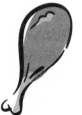

Poultry: Lean And Mean

POULTRY IS A PIECE OF CAKE — well, you know what we mean. It's just easy to figure out, because the fat lives in the skin. Take that off, and what's left is lean. If you want the leanest possible, use kitchen scissors to trim off the little globs or streaks of fat that cling to the chicken once the skin has been taken off. On the other hand, if you deep-fry chicken, or if you cover it with a cheese or cream sauce, low fat goes out the window. Ditto for prepared chicken that you find in a foil tray in the freezer section of the super-market. Healthiest is baked or broiled, and if you want a sauce, make it tomato. Delicious.

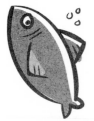 ### Sat Fat Worry-Free: Fish

FISH IS PART OF THE "MEAT/POULTRY GROUP," which now becomes, obviously, the "meat/poul-try/fish group." The three go together because they are all good sources of protein. But fish is a differ-ent, well, a different kettle of fish. Yes, it contains protein, but, unlike meat and poultry, fat is not an issue. You may have heard rumors that fish is fatty, and some fish are (salmon, for example), but the fat in fish is healthy. This good fat is known as "omega-3," a name perhaps better suited to be the title of a Tom Clancy novel. It is, however, a fat that is particularly protective for your heart.

Eating fish may very well be the easiest way to reduce the risk of heart disease. Only if a fish is deep fried or otherwise cooked in a lot of fat is it the kind of "fatty" you'll want to avoid. Otherwise, eat a vari-ety of fish, and you'll get a variety of benefits. Include all fish, shell-fish, too, which is very low in fat. Enjoy it occasionally; there is no rea-son to avoid it, unless, of course, there are other reasons why you should not eat it. You don't have to eat large amounts of fish, either. Just two meals a week, with a serving size of 3 ounces at each meal, will do the trick, an amount that will be, by now, a familiar quantity.

The recommendation to eat fish more frequently is really nothing new. But maybe you harbor a lingering resentment because of all those Fridays when you had to eat fish. Or maybe you really dislike the idea of extra trips to the food store to buy fish — which, admit-tedly, doesn't keep very long. It will keep longer if you put the pack-age in a bowl filled with ice cubes before putting it in the refrigerator.

Nothing tastes as good as really fresh fish, which you'll want to buy from a place that sells a lot of it, keeps it on ice, and sees to it that what you are getting does not have a fishy smell. Some frozen versions run a close second to fresh these days. So if for whatever reason fresh is not available, try frozen, but please, not fish sticks. They are "fish-like," maybe, but that's it. (Besides, chances are that

THE HEALTHY WEIGH: Eat fish at least twice a week, but NOT fish sandwiches at fast food places.

the breading has a lot of fat in it, the very thing you're trying to avoid.) Your supermarket freezer section has different types of frozen fish, and new and improved packaging for it. Now sealed in clear plastic wrap, you can actually see what you are buying. Worth a try, because this fish will likely taste better than the frozen fish in your past.

There is another alternative to fresh fish, and that is canned, yes, canned, convenient and easy to keep on hand. Needs no refrigeration, either. You're most familiar with canned tuna, but consider salmon. You might want to start with Chicken of the Sea pink salmon, which is very much like tuna, and therefore offers the pleasure of the familiar. Then you might move on and try red salmon, which has quite a different (and wonderful!) taste. Most canned salmon has the extra added attraction of bones, which fall apart easily as you mash them up, providing you with a nice source of calcium.

Canned salmon has a certain allure. Keep it on your shelf and it will be ready, willing, and able to jump in when guests arrive unexpectedly and food reinforcements are called for. You'll be serving something that is beautiful and tasty, and, maybe best of all, looks like you put in a lot more work than you really did. It is truly a best-kept secret. Use it as an appetizer on crackers, in a salad, or as a main course. Works for everything but dessert.

For its fish oils and its delicious flavor, salmon deserves an award for versatility and desirability in the fish world. And its own limerick.

A FISH STORY

The versatile salmon is great
In a salad or just on a plate.
Whether fresh or in cans,
It has numerous fans,
And omega-3's make it first-rate.

Now that is a story worth telling,
And salmon is certainly selling.
It's a wonderful fish –
Makes a wonderful dish –
The only thing strange is its spelling.

CHANGE OF PACE

NOW THAT YOU KNOW you can eat meat, poultry, and fish, the only thing left to do is to eat all of them. Over the course of a week, though, not all at once. And in 3-ounce servings, too. Different foods offer different benefits, and you'll see that the "14-Day Meal Plan with Meal Appeal" includes a variety of foods.

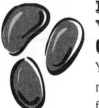

More Sat Fat Worry-Free: Beans (a.k.a. "Legumes")

YOU MAY BE USED TO getting your protein from meat, poultry, and fish. Take another step away from sat fat. Welcome to the wonderful world of beans. They offer a pleasant change of pace, so one day when you find yourself in the supermarket idly wondering when they'll invent a new meat, try beans. They come in bags and cans, making them easy to store, and they'll keep for a long, long time. And now for something new: Edamame, packaged by Seaside Farms, Cascadian Farms, and others, are delicious frozen soybeans that cook in a few minutes in boiling water. It just doesn't come any easier. Besides the obvious health benefits, you'll love the fact that, as long as you've prepared these foods with an eye toward health (no cream, no butter, no cheese), you don't need to worry about fat. Low fat and loving it.

You might like to go non-meat several times a week, or maybe every day of the week, a vegetarian diet. This offers extra opportunities to eat vegetables, whole grains, and fruits, always a good idea.

THE HEALTHY WEIGH: Have a vegetarian meal at least once a week.

A POSTHUMOUS COLLABORATION

ELVIS HAS COME BACK FROM THE DEAD (assuming you believe he's dead, and if you don't — well, the collaboration isn't posthumous, is it?) to help us with a song to sum things up. Here it is, courtesy of "The King."

ARE YOU FAMISHED TONIGHT?

(Tune: "Are You Lonesome Tonight?")

Are you famished tonight?
Are you famished tonight?
Are you sorry you can't eat much fat?
Does your memory stray
To your porterhouse days,
When your steak was the size of a mat?
Does your vegetable platter seem overly bland?
Do your beans, rice, and pasta seem overly planned?
Is your heart filled with pain?
(Not if you're eating grain!)
Tell me, dear, are you famished tonight?

IN A NUTSHELL:
Start today! Instead of meat, have fish for dinner.

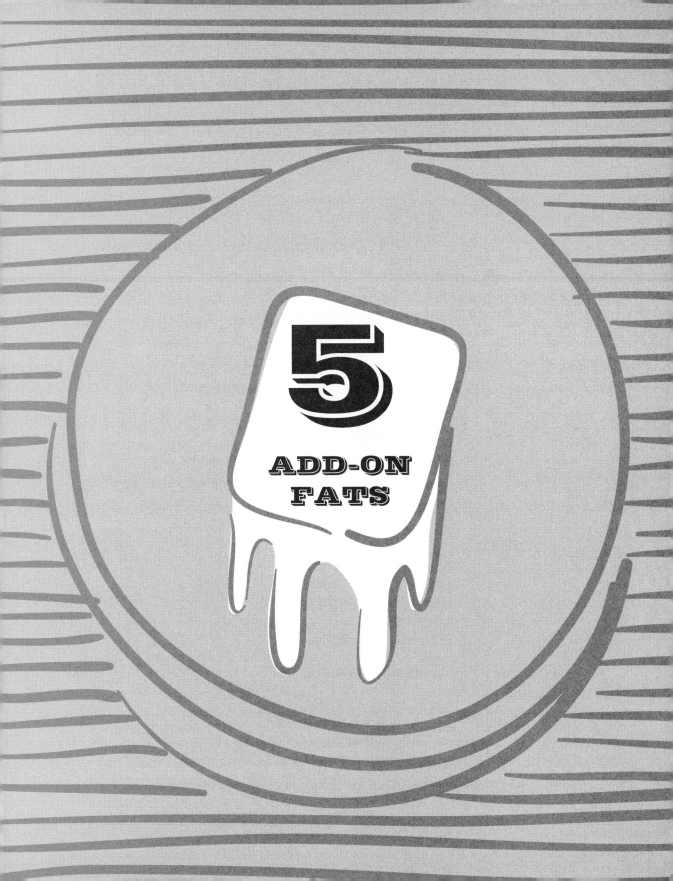

5

ADD-ON FATS

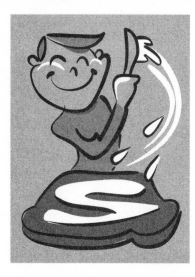

WE'VE SPENT A LOT OF TIME talking about dairy, meat, and poultry, foods that contain fat, and, most importantly, sat fat. Nature put it in there, but you don't have to have it. For your health, get the sat fat level down with "low-fat" (or "lean") versions. ★ Then there are add-on sat fats — butter, cream cheese, sour cream. Nature doesn't add them to the food, you do. Don't. Read on.

FATS WITH A GOOD REPUTATION

SAT FAT IS NOT THE ONLY FAT, but it is the one with the worst reputation. ★ Fats from plants, however, have a reputation that sat fat would die for. At the opposite end of the fats spectrum, these fats are called *un*saturated. You may know that olive oil and canola oil are prime examples. Those who live in Mediterranean countries have known the secret of these oils for a long time, use olive oil (monounsaturated) in their cooking, and enjoy its health benefits. Canola oil doesn't have the history of olive oil, but it may well have the promise. Other plants that provide nice oils are safflower, sunflower, corn, sesame, and soy. (These are, by the way, often used to make mayonnaise, salad dressing, and margarine.) If you are confused about what fat to use in cooking, you may want to go with any of these oils, but go easy: about one teaspoon added fat per serving. One teaspoon of oil on a plate is about the size of a quarter. Doesn't sound like much, but a little goes a long way.

Good fat comes in many forms. There are some that might not strike you as being fats, but surprise, surprise! They are. Think olives and avocados, seeds and nuts (including peanut butter, a spreadable nut). Here's an interesting tidbit: "Nuts" spelled backwards is "stun," and you may be stunned to discover that nuts really are good for you. Still, like everything else on this list, they are add-IN fats, and so you'll want to add them (sparingly) to your food. Don't work your way through a jar of nuts and call it dinner.

THE HEALTHY WEIGH: Plant fats are good for you.

PLANTS AND SCIENCE: A STRUGGLING RELATIONSHIP

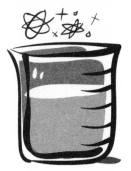

NOTHING IS PERFECT, and it turns out that plant fats can be transformed, making them hazardous to your health. Unfortunately they have no warning labels. Ah, the wonders of modern science! A chemical process known as hydrogenation takes a poor, unsuspecting vegetable oil and changes it so that it becomes solid and spreadable (margarine, shortening), and lengthens the shelf life of the products it is found in. Good idea? No, bad idea, because the process results in the creation of not only sat fat, but also "trans fat," which mimics the effect of saturated fats on the body. They are the "gruesome twosome" when it comes to dangerous fats. You don't need any saturated fat in your diet, and you certainly don't need a cheap imitation.

Trans fat turns out to be at least as harmful as saturated fat and is found in (hard to spell much less pronounce) hydrogenated and partially hydrogenated oils. Because it doesn't spoil, this disreputable fat is found in most margarines and in processed foods —

crackers, chips, and other snack foods; cookies and other commercially baked goods. It's all over the place. Whether you know it or not, you're getting a lot of trans fat if you spend any time at all in fast food restaurants, because it's in the oils used for cooking, frying — even baking hamburger rolls.

How do you know if there is trans fat in the food you buy at the supermarket? As of this writing, you don't. Even when the food carries a Nutrition Facts label, you don't, because the words "trans fat" appear nowhere on the ingredient list or in Nutrition Facts. You have to be a regular Sherlock Holmes, sleuthing your way along. You deduce the fact that trans fat is in there because, as we've just said, it is found in hydrogenated and partially hydrogenated oils, which are listed in the ingredients.

We've been hearing for some time now that "soon" Nutrition Facts will be sporting new information. That is, the FDA has proposed that trans fat be added to saturated fat on the label. When this comes to pass, an asterisk (or some yet-undisclosed symbol) after "saturated fat" will most likely direct you to a footnote at the bottom of the label, where you'll see the amount of trans fat in the food.

We live in a toxic food environment, and it's just not possible to know where all the trans fat is. We're told by the National Academy of Sciences to cut back on trans fat, but how can we if we don't know it's there? So what's the answer? Go with the best foods on earth! They are as low in trans fat as you can get.

THE HEALTHY WEIGH:

Stay away from trans fat.

FATS & WEIGHT LOSS

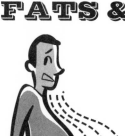

FATS ARE FATTENING. There is really compelling evidence that successful weight loss depends on low fat. (Want to see the "compelling evidence"? Check the Endnotes under "Weight Loss.") Fats add up quickly, more quickly than other foods. Tidbit: You could eat one tablespoon of mayonnaise and it would be equal, gaining-weight-wise, to a baked potato and an apple. You get less bang for the buck with fats than with anything else. By the way — one tablespoon of margarine or mayonnaise is about the size of a ping pong ball. If your fat doesn't keep a nice shape and spreads around, like oil, then one tablespoon is about the size of a teabag.

A LOW-FAT DAY

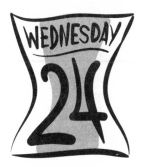

LET'S LOOK AT WHAT A LOW-FAT DAY is all about. Essentially, it's a little bit of add-on fat with every meal. If you keep track, not only will you be healthier, you will also be far less likely to gain weight.

Breakfast first. On your English muffin, put 2 teaspoons of margarine or 4 teaspoons of peanut butter. You're already having low-fat milk with your cereal, and a piece of fruit as well. That's because you've read the beginning of this book.

Lunch. On your salad, put 2 tablespoons of regular salad dressing or 4 tablespoons of low-fat dressing, and add some cut-up fruit. Try honey mustard instead of mayonnaise for a great spread on your grilled chicken breast sandwich.

Dinner. Sauté your mixed vegetables in 2 teaspoons of olive oil. Next to your baked potato with fat-free sour cream, put a piece of broiled salmon (yippee! Omega-3!). Finish with a piece of fruit and a glass of low-fat milk.

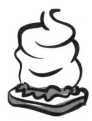

Stumbling Blocks to a Low-Fat Day

SO — HOW ARE YOU DOING? Having a low-fat day? Not if your lunchtime sandwich was tuna salad made with regular old mayonnaise. Startling news: If you made your tuna salad with only two *level* tablespoons of mayonnaise (highly unlikely), *that one sandwich has the same amount of fat you would have gotten in the entire low-fat day described a minute ago.* Chances are you used considerably more than two tablespoons of mayo, and, if you bought your tuna salad sandwich rather than made it at home, it most definitely had a whole lot more.

There are other stumbling blocks. When you buy salads at a take-out place, they tend to have an awful lot of dressing, making them a higher-fat food than you realize. If you cook with margarine and use a whole stick, keep in mind you are using 24 teaspoons, which is enough to float in. That much fat is frying, pure and simple, and fried anything adds more fat than you want.

LABELS: KEEPING TRACK OF FAT IN PACKAGED FOODS

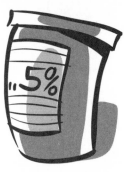

SO YOU'VE SEEN HOW TO DEAL with add-on fats. Now you'll want to know how to deal with the fat in packaged foods, and labels give you a shot at doing that. How? By telling you quickly and easily whether or not you should even consider buying a given item.

The key to choosing low fat is a bold percentage to the right of the words "**Total Fat**." This is "**% Daily Value**." You can use this to see if your food has a small amount of something — 5% or less (you don't want much fat) — or a large amount of something — 20% or more (you want a larger amount of fiber). *Look for 5% OR LESS DAILY VALUE FOR TOTAL FAT.*

	% Daily Value*
Total Fat 3g	**5%**

That is a small amount of fat per serving.

There is one teensy-weensy little thing. **Serving Size**. You really have to pay attention, because *everything else on the label is based on it*. It's just that the serving size on the label doesn't necessarily bear much resemblance to the amount you, personally, eat. You'll need to think Own Personal Serving Size — OPSS — when reading a label. How big is your serving? Compare it to the one on the label and you may find that you have some calculating to do. If you eat two or three times the amount that the label calls a serving, then **% Daily Value** will have to be multiplied by two or three or whatever. It doesn't take much to go from OPSS to OOPS!

Now maybe you're savvy, savvy enough to have found a nice, low-fat cookie that just suits your personality. You knew it at a glance. You looked at the Total Fat and saw that, for a serving size of two cookies, % Daily Value is 5%. You do know how to read labels! So you're sitting with the crossword puzzle and a glass of milk and your low-fat cookies. Two. Then three, then four, then five, then — who knows how many? If that "who knows how many?" was ten cookies, your % Daily Value was five times 5%, or 25% of the day's fat in just those ten little cookies. Like a magic trick, before your very eyes, low fat became high fat. You went from OPSS to OOPS!

LOW FAT BECOMES SECOND NATURE

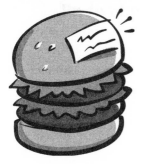 LABELS CAN ONLY DO SO MUCH. Besides, a lot of the food you eat doesn't come in bags or boxes or any other package. You cook, you eat out, you live a life that is largely label free. Eventually you will become so familiar with how things fit together that you will understand the relative place of fat in the diet. You'll know which cuts of meat are lowest in fat, and that you don't need to eat much of them. An appealing fringe benefit will be that you'll feel better when there is less fat in your diet, and you'll very likely come to the point where you and fatty foods are not so attracted to each other anymore. Tastes do change. Give your tastebuds a chance. You're worth it.

THE HEALTHY WEIGH: Keep a lid on fat and serving size.

IN A NUTSHELL:
Start today! Make a dinner with no packaged or processed foods at all.

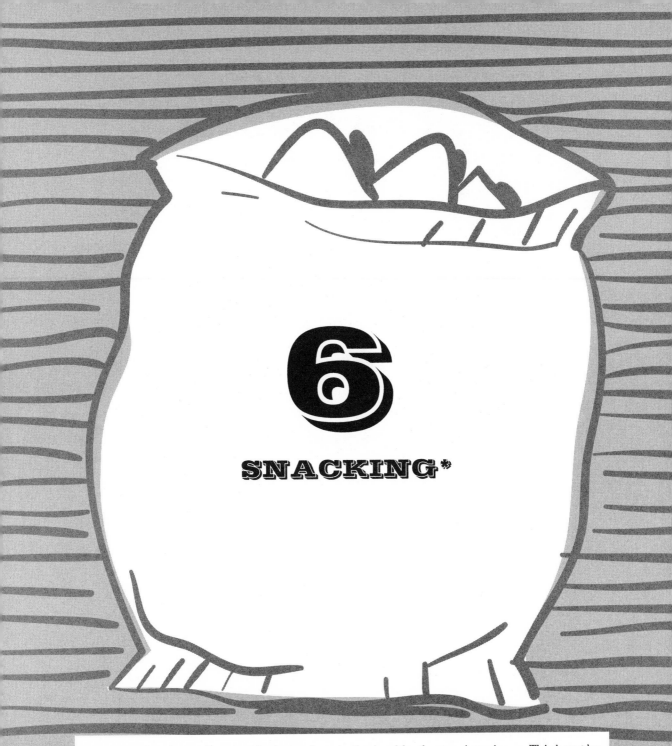

6

SNACKING*

*Snacking has been shown to be hazardous to the health of many Americans. Think you're an exception? Check with your doctor. Together you can determine whether or not this chapter is relevant to you in particular.

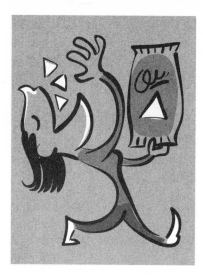

EATING MEALS INSTEAD OF SNACKING

WHAT ARE YOU DOING that increases your likelihood of snacking? ① Not planning breakfast, lunch, dinner ② Not eating breakfast, lunch, dinner ③ Not eating well-balanced meals ④ Not allowing enough time for meals (planning goes out the window) ★ What can you do to decrease your likelihood of snacking? Eat MEALS — yes, just like Mom used to tell you. (Do the words "You'll spoil your dinner!" mean anything to you?) You won't find yourself ravenous at some point during the day or evening if you have broken up your waking hours with three good, filling meals. You want them to be "good" and "filling," because it's possible to eat three skimpy, poorly balanced meals every day and feel unsatisfied all the time. But wait, you persist, what can I do? I snack because I am really hungry! ★ Are you sure your meals are filling you up? Are you eating enough food? Does your plate look full and beautiful? You want your answer to be a resounding "yes" to all these questions.

You can eat a lot, feel pleasantly satisfied, and not gain weight *if you choose the right foods*. If you want to feel satisfied, you have to eat enough food. Quantity counts. The way to eat enough food without gaining weight is easy. Picture a plate of pasta, for example, a reasonable serving. Might look a little skimpy. Now picture that same amount of pasta combined with beautifully cooked vegetables and a fresh tomato sauce. The plate will be full and so will you.

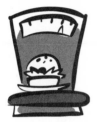

Odd Thought For Today

STUDIES HAVE SHOWN that people are hardwired to eat a certain weight of food each day in order to be satisfied (that is, filled up). We can actually measure the weight of the food eaten on a daily basis and show that *people eat about the same weight of food every day.*

We know that different foods have different weights and different calorie content. What you are looking for is food that weighs a lot but doesn't have a lot of calories. Adding those vegetables to the pasta a minute ago added weight but not calories. See how it works?

SNACKING: GETTING THE BEST BANG FOR THE BUCK

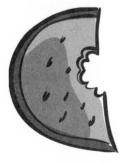

LET'S SAY you are eating good meals (really, we believe you if you say you are doing that) but are still hungry. What do you do? Something that Mom probably told you never to do — eat between meals. In other words, have snacks. Like meals, they should be satisfying (plenty of food) but not loaded with calories. After all, you're not trying to gain weight. Or are you?

Try this. Which would make a more filling snack, half a watermelon or a handful of jelly candies (which, by the way, are equivalent calorie-wise)? All together now: the watermelon! It gives you the best bang for the buck, or B for the B, because you get to eat much

THE HEALTHY WEIGH: You want to make your meal look like you are eating a lot of food, but without a lot of calories. You feel more satisfied. If you don't know how to do this, here's an example: Add a cup of vegetables to a cup of pasta. Two cups of food for the calorie price of one!

**THE
HEALTHY WEIGH:**
Think "satisfaction,"
and choose foods that
fill you up without a lot
of calories — fruits,
vegetables, low-fat
dairy, and whole
grains.

**THE
HEALTHY WEIGH:**
Your new definition of
a snack: A snack is an
opportunity to get in
the fruits, vegetables,
low-fat dairy, and
whole grains that you
didn't have in your
three meals.

**THE
HEALTHY WEIGH:**
Limit sugary foods.

more food for the same calorie price. The foods that give you the best B for the B, for meals and for snacks, are — you're way ahead of us — fruits, vegetables, low-fat dairy, and whole grains. The best diet on earth.

Snacks: An Opportunity

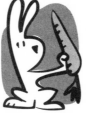

NOW YOU HAVE AN OPPORTUNITY to eat the fruits, vegetables, low-fat dairy, and whole grains that you didn't have in your three meals. Try filling up with something like a bowl of cereal with low-fat milk. Or have some whole grains — low-fat microwave popcorn is a good choice, as are baked corn tortilla chips. Try fruit and milk together. It's filling and tasty and a healthier combo than cookies and milk (if not as Santa-sounding).

SNACKING AS WE KNOW IT

A LOT OF SOCIAL ACTIVITY in this country is based on snacking. We "meet and eat," if not for a meal, then for a quasi-meal, maybe pie and coffee. Back in elementary school, snacking was our favorite "subject." In high school, dates included snacking. When our kids were young, we had snacking opportunities galore with our friends while our kids played together. Snacking is the American way.

So what exactly is "snacking"? You probably know it when you see it, have some sense that it involves eating from bags and boxes, but read on. Definition (ours, not Webster's): Snacking is a repeated, mindless, food event that has little, if anything, to do with hunger. It is an activity, a pastime, maybe even a hobby. It involves the ingestion of either quasi-food-like substances known for their high caloric content and low food value, or actual food eaten to excess.

Say you sit down in front of the TV with a pint of "Loco Cocoa Mocho" ice cream, ready to watch a "Friends" re-run. You come to at the end of the show and notice the ice cream is among the missing. You have no recollection of eating it, but you're home alone and the dog is asleep. Sound like a fit? No? What, you don't like "Friends," or you don't eat ice cream? Okay, make it A&E "Biography" and baked corn chips with salsa. M-m-m-m. Healthy. Now "Biography" comes on, a pretty good one, maybe Grace Kelly, and then it's over and so is the bag of corn chips. And the salsa. Tomorrow night, same thing. Well, not Grace Kelly. You could call this a hobby, but probably not one you'd care to include on your resume. It's also a lot of calories you're gathering together, and you will gain weight.

SUSPICIOUS HEALTH MESSAGES

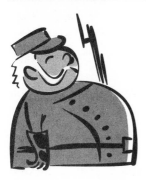

FREQUENT EATING FOR HEALTH has a long history. Back in the days of the Civil War, underweight people were fed 26 times a day. When you stop and think that they were asleep for part of each 24-hour day, those 26 feedings really took up a lot of time. Underweight was considered a serious health problem back then, whereas a hefty weight was thought to be a mark of robust health. (Times do change, don't they?) This is proof positive — as if we needed it — that frequent eating helps people gain weight.

With all we know today about snacking and weight gain, it's ironic that the message to snack originally came as a health message. But the fact that certain medical conditions can be helped by having frequent snacks has exploded in the marketplace and has become . . . (drum roll) . . . the SNACKING INDUSTRY. Snack food manufacturers are not deaf. They are listening to the health messages out there and are acting accordingly. If there's a way to ride the crest of a health message and boost sales, they'll do it. Low fat is good for your health? Low-fat and fat-free snack foods come to market. Some people shouldn't have sugar? Sugar-free snack foods

> **THE HEALTHY WEIGH:** If you're gaining weight, look at snacking. And if you're gaining weight, be on the lookout for high blood pressure, diabetes, and high cholesterol.

emerge. Some people shouldn't have salt? Here come the low-sodi-um and sodium-free snack foods. Need energy? Energy bars or ener-gy drinks. (And yes, drinks can be snack "foods." Have a soda and you're having a snack drink. Sorry, but that's the reality.) The last frontier — whole grain snack foods. We're betting they're on the way. Just watch.

Today, people are being bombarded by advertisements for snack food and by its availability, seduced into the behavior we call snack-ing. And it's working. Surveys show that people are snacking more than ever. Manufacturers play with your palate using taste (sweet, salty) and smell (um-m-m) the minute you open a package. There is new and easier-than-ever access to snack foods in unexpected places. Vending machines are now found in schools (is it any won-der kids eat what's in there?), and they sit outside of some highway rest stops so you can save yourself the trouble of walking through the door. Office supply stores have gigantic, conference-size packages of snack foods, the containers for which can double as trash baskets. Then there are the more obvious places. Convenience stores are par-ticularly convenient for snack foods.

Super-availablility is, of course, in the supermaket. Just check out the snack food aisles (how many varieties of chips can there be?) and see, in real life, what the many, many television ads have been hawking. With snack food companies behind them all the way, peo-ple are snacking too much. That serves the snack food industry well. It is getting bigger by making people bigger, because bigger people eat more.

THE HEALTHY WEIGH: Americans are getting fatter. According to RAND research on the health risks of obesity, one in five is obese; three in five are either overweight or obese.

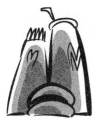

Super Sizing: Our Toxic Food Environment

WHY TOXIC? Because it means "poisonous, lethal, deadly, contaminated," and this food environment is hazardous to your health. Portion sizes are getting bigger, and so are we. In 1970, portion sizes began to grow and are still growing. As an example, old and new editions of classic cookbooks (The Joy of Cooking, for instance) show the same recipe for cookies in both editions, but with one striking change — recipes in the newer editions serve fewer people. This means that each serving is bigger than it used to be. Restaurants are using bigger plates to accommodate bigger portions. Even home dinner plates are now bigger than ever. If you buy a new set of dishes, don't be surprised if they don't fit in your dishwasher.

A researcher with a keen eye, a food scale, and manufacturer's information compared the sizes of common snack foods past and present. It used to be that there was no choice in the size of chocolate bars, french fries, and sodas. Now there are various sizes to choose from, the smallest of which is the same size as, or bigger than, the old original size. Sizing and re-sizing is big these days. Women's clothing is being "vanity sized," since it became clear that women like to think they fit into small sizes. They don't, but apparently that's beside the point. Manufacturers simply did a little re-numbering, so if you used to wear a size 12, suddenly, magically, you are wearing a size 10.

McDonald's is re-numbering in order to increase sales. The 1998 "Supersize" soda was re-named "Large" in 2001. We live in a toxic food environment, and food is being sized to make us bigger. Don't ask us how big the Supersize is now — or the projected size in 2010. Suffice it to say, it will come with a truss.

Maybe the toxic snack food environment is beyond your control, but only you can turn snack food into snacking. (And only you can prevent forest fires. Smokey thanks you for being careful.) You can control the "mindless event," the repetition, the choice of foods, and if you can't, you need a snack therapist.

THE HEALTHY WEIGH:
Downsize your foods.

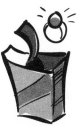

Fun Food: the Toxic Food Environment, continued

IT'S NO SURPRISE that the snacking industry is on the "let's have fun!" bandwagon. It began with Cracker Jack and the prizes inside, and has moved on to playful packaging, even playful sizes, like bite-size Oreos (to cite one example), geared for little hands to hold.

That's snack food. When did regular old food become "fun"? Breakfast cereals have been fun for a long time, what with games on the back of the boxes, and prizes inside. Every kid saved box tops to send in for special goodies, too. You'll notice, however, that the fun did not involve the food itself. What happened? It seems to us that colored cereals, some with marshmallows, led the way, back when our children were children. Now we've gone to an extreme. Unless food is fun — and parents want their kids to have fun — the kids won't eat it.

What was once just nourishing food now has to be entertaining — yes, entertaining. Think of yogurt, good and healthy. Well, now it comes sweeter than ever, with a "side" of sprinkle-on crunchies. Yogurt also comes in a tube, so that you can suck it. Fun, huh? It also comes in colors, if you please, even glow-in-the-dark. Must be for the kids who are playing in the closet while they are eating their yogurt.

And they do like to play when they're eating, don't they? Maybe it's TV or Game Boy with dinner. They've been trained by fun meals, Happy Meals, where toys and food go hand-in-hand. Fun food comes home (or goes to school) in the form of "lunchables," little plastic containers with a couple of crackers, a little hunk of cheese, a bit of meat, and — the reason for buying this in the first place — a toy.

So what's the connection between "toxic food environment" and fun food? Here's the bad news: you can't make good food choices when fun is a concern. It's just not possible. Food is delicious, beautiful, wonderful, pleasurable, etc., etc., etc., but fun? No. Food is food, and fun is fun. Occasionally they meet (fondue /"fun-do," making candy apples), but when they meet too often, you're in a toxic food environment.

SNAX TAX

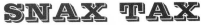

WHAT WE NEED is a National Snacking Reform Policy. How about warning labels on snack foods? "Warning: Snacking may be hazardous to your health"? How about curbs on advertising? How about taxing snack foods — a "snax tax"? Anything that affects national health needs special funding to support the costs associated with health problems that develop as a result of use. Why not a tax? They did it for cigarettes. Believe it or not, it costs more to take care of the health problems of an obese person than of a cigarette smoker. So why not pay attention to the cost of obesity in America? "$Paying attention$" — you can take it literally. A snax tax can help cut down the rate of obesity, just the way cigarette and alcohol taxes have helped reduce the rates of smoking and drinking. Same thing goes for curbs on advertising.

IT'S UP TO YOU

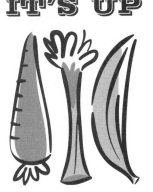

IDEALLY, SNACKING AS WE KNOW IT disappears from the planet. What we are left with is three healthy, satisfying meals. And what happens if you are hungry between meals? You have something to eat — maybe a piece of fruit, or a glass of milk, or both. Or maybe whole grains (slice of whole wheat toast). You've already seen how to use food for the good of your body, and that fruits, vegetables, low-fat dairy, and whole grains pack a real health wallop. Now you know your snack can do the same thing. A snack is an opportunity to get in the fruits, vegetables, low-fat dairy, and whole grains that you didn't have in your three meals. The old snacking involved "extras," adding foods that you might not eat at a meal. This doesn't. Besides, if you eat well-balanced meals, you'll be less likely to snack.

THE HEALTHY WEIGH: Less snacking can mean weight loss! Do the math: If your daily trip to the convenience store also includes snacking, you may be able to lose weight just by not snacking. If you change your pattern and not get that snack cake every day, you could lose up to 1 pound a week. We know someone who discovered that he was over 200 pounds, stopped snacking, and got himself down to his former fighting weight of 180. "The No Ding-Dong Diet" he calls it.

Wouldn't it be nice if there was the same kind of blockbuster advertising money behind fruits and vegetables, low-fat dairy, and whole grains, so they could compete with snack foods? Imagine — "'E.R.', brought to you by broccoli."

IN A NUTSHELL:

Start today! If you are hungry between meals, have a piece of fruit and a slice of whole grain toast. Really hungry? Add a glass of low-fat or fat-free milk.

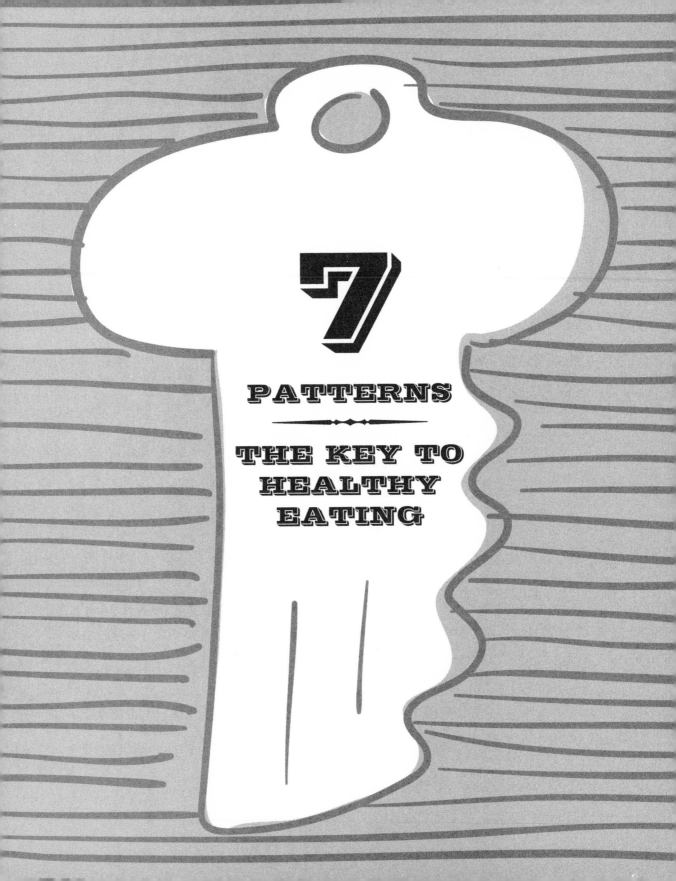

7

PATTERNS

THE KEY TO HEALTHY EATING

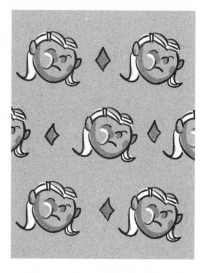

YOU KNOW PATTERNS; you have many patterns in your life. You walk, you get hiccups, you have a favorite plaid scarf. You sew, you knit. You play golf and tennis, and you learn patterns of stroking the ball. You love square dancing. You drive the same way to work every day. You have male-pattern baldness. You have a menstrual cycle. Your life has patterns. ★ Patterns occur over and over again. That's what makes them patterns in the first place — the ability to be replicated. Some patterns are better than others. Some patterns are in your control. The ones we talk about in this chapter are definitely in your control. They are your food patterns, the way food fits into your day. There are things you can do to improve those patterns, and we're going to examine them together. ★ The question is, where do you start? First you have to know where you are. (That would be what you are eating, not where you live.) So where are you? What do you eat in the way of fruits, vegetables, low-fat dairy, and whole grains on a given day? We're not asking what you think you should eat, but what you actually *do* eat in a day.

DOWN MEMORY LANE

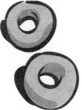

Discovering Your Own Personal Food Pattern

IN ORDER TO FIGURE THIS OUT, let's take a walk down Memory Lane (it's a short walk, just the last 24 hours) and think about everything you had to eat. No fair developing an instant case of food amnesia or a sudden attack of guilt. Maybe you stopped for a Krispy Kreme or two or three on the way to work. You may have had fast food for lunch and dinner. Maybe there's an irresistible candy dish at work. The point here is simply to remember, and to remember accurately, which you can do if you try. Don't be surprised if your trip down Memory Lane is uncomfortable. You're going to learn a lot about yourself. You might not eat as many fruits and vegetables as you think you do. You might find you skip meals more than you realized. You're learning about your eating style.

Also, there are practical matters in trying to remember, since days have a way of blending together. "Was it yesterday or the day before that we went out for pizza?" A simple way to solve this practical problem is to break up the day into pieces. This makes it easier to see a pattern. Let's do that now, starting with larger pieces, and let's call them "breakfast," "lunch," and "dinner." Not original, maybe, but useful nevertheless. It may help to think about where you had those meals and if there was anything special about them.

Breakfast: Where were you and what did you have? By the way — was there any fruit involved? Vegetables? Any milk?

Lunch: Ditto

Dinner: Ditto

Now consider the day's record. What's your eating style? Wait, you protest, this was an unusual day! I don't usually eat this way! This was a quirky day! Well, look at more days and you'll get a more accurate picture.

Suppose you are someone who feels your life is too complex to allow you the luxury of dividing the day into large pieces called "meals," that you have no pattern at all. You might think patterns are just plain rigid. If you eat whenever you feel like it and figure you don't need meals, your trip down Memory Lane will be a more diffi-

THE HEALTHY WEIGH: If you want to lose weight, keep a food record. Write down exactly what and how much you eat, and do it immediately after eating. Be honest. Keep good records.

cult one, maybe too difficult. If this is the case, instead of going down Memory Lane, try going forward in time. It will be easier if you write everything down, not just think about it. This is your food record. Not bestseller material, but worthwhile nonetheless. (See pages 138-140 for the you-fill-in Food Records at the back of this book.)

Maybe your morning involves stopping at a convenience store every morning for a headlight-size muffin, eating a fast food lunch in the car, and having a late dinner standing at the kitchen counter and eating by the light of the open refrigerator door. By writing everything down for a whole day — better yet, for three days — you'll know exactly what you ate on a given day, as well as when you ate it, and whether or not you included fruits, vegetables, low-fat dairy, and whole grains.. (By the way, if your records look too good, you might be under-reporting, which is not uncommon.)

When you look at your honest record, even though you have no regular meals to form a pattern, and even though you think patterns are rigid, look! You have one after all, and not a very healthy one at that. Now your job will be to replace one pattern for another — healthy for not-so-healthy.

A HEALTHY PATTERN: THREE MEALS A DAY

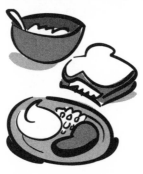

FIRST YOU'RE GOING TO have to plan to eat meals, set aside distinct periods of time during the day when you focus on eating the food that will satisfy your appetite. We know you're already satisfying your appetite — it's all the rage. Everybody's doing it. The idea is to provide yourself with those "distinct periods of time" — otherwise known as breakfast, lunch, and dinner. Three meals a day may seem a little old-fashioned, but they serve as markers to remind you to eat, and they give you the opportunity to eat well. After all, meals are your best chance to eat fruits, vegetables, low-fat dairy, and whole grains, so it is, quite simply, eas-

THE HEALTHY WEIGH:
If weight loss is part of your healthy weigh but you're not losing weight, you need a better understanding of what you're really eating. Keep a three day food record and get out those measuring spoons and a food scale.

ier to be healthy if you eat breakfast, lunch, and dinner. What if you don't eat three meals? Your day lacks the kind of orderliness that leads to success — that is, healthy eating.

You may eat only two meals on any given day, for whatever reason. Maybe you'd rather "sleep in" that extra fifteen minutes than eat breakfast, or work through lunch, or go directly to the mall after work instead of home for dinner, and not get home until bedtime. On those days when you skip a meal (we bet that meal is most often breakfast), it's harder to get the healthy stuff worked in, because you've now eliminated one-third of the day's opportunities for doing that. (Through no fault of their own this commonly happens to shift workers — policemen, firemen, nurses — who, while taking care of us, find themselves in a situation where it's very difficult to take care of themselves. We'll address this later on.)

To repeat: Breakfast, lunch, and dinner are where the fruits, vegetables, low-fat dairy, and whole grains are found. Give yourself a break, and go for the Big Three.

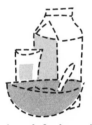

Pattern: Breakfast, The Endangered Species

PEOPLE ARE NOT EATING BREAKFAST. As Americans are losing their interest in this important meal, breakfast is becoming an endangered species, which is a shame, since it doesn't have to be traditional. It doesn't have to be big and hearty (good news if you really don't like the idea of eating breakfast in the first place), and "breakfast foods" can be anything that's good and wholesome. Worth noting — breakfast-eaters tend to have the advantage when it comes to the rest of the day, because, as a group, they eat less fat, more vitamins and minerals, and they weigh less than non-breakfast-eaters. Surprised? Maybe you skip breakfast because you are trying to lose weight and have resolved to eat less. Doesn't work like that, though, since the rest of the day more than makes up for the skipped meal. Oh — did we mention that breakfast-eaters are smarter, scoring better on tests? AND they have more energy? Wouldn't you like to join this prestigious group? A possible bumper sticker: "Breakfast + Grains = Brains." Now *that's* an equation.

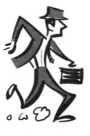

Pattern: In a Hurry, Breakfast and Lunch

IN TOO MUCH OF A HURRY TO EAT BREAKFAST? Lunch hour slipping by and you haven't eaten? Join the crowd — everybody seems to be in a hurry these days — but "in a hurry" doesn't have to mean "eating poorly."

You've stopped for gas on the way to work, and you run into the quickie mart to refuel yourself. Your breakfast. Note that these stores don't specialize in breakfast foods, but you are going to develop a new pattern and find suitable breakfast foods, suitable for eating in the car (your eatery of choice). You can get a balanced breakfast at the quickie mart. Get some string cheese or yogurt or milk (low fat or fat free), and half a bagel (no cream cheese). Then bypass the doughnut, cookie, and chips shelves and head straight for the fruit section. You will be delighted at the quality of the individual fruits sold at this unexpected "fruit stand," sometimes even at very good prices. And always convenient. When was the last time you had someone cut up your fresh fruit? Remember ice cream sundae cups? These are already filled — not with ice cream, but with fruit. You can buy whole fruit, any fruit, we don't care. Just buy some fruit.

While you're at it, pick up lunch at the same time. Get your lunchtime fruit ("fruit at every meal"). If you've calculated correctly, you have half a bagel left over from breakfast, a bagel that was actually big enough to serve two. Take the other half with you for lunch. And see if there's a nice salad, all packaged and ready to go. Add yogurt, and there's lunch.

No time to stop at the quickie mart? Sounds like you're on your way to a fast food restaurant. What is there to say? Jay Leno says that at McDonald's, when you order fries, they say, "Do you want fries with that?"

At fast food places they have drive-thru windows, which works out nicely if you're in a car. And you will be, won't you? Because you're in hurry. Your new pattern is milk, juice, and broiled chicken or a junior (not a misprint) hamburger. If you don't want to drink both juice and milk, try to have a piece of fruit with you. You'll have some if you've put together a Car Emergency Kit, things to keep in your car: small box of raisins; juice box; flip-top can of fruit. Oh, yes — and a few plastic spoons. Put it all in a zip-lock bag with a napkin or two. Meeting run late? Traffic backed up? This will help you out at lunchtime — or anytime — and keep you from being famished when you get to your food destination.

If you're lucky enough to have time to go inside the fast food place, you can get a salad, which wouldn't have been so easy to eat in the car. You won't be inside very long, because the seat backs are specially designed to be slightly uncomfortable so you won't hang around.

The atmosphere is nothing to write home about, but you can improve lunchtime ambiance by bringing a lunch from home and eating it while you sit outside on a nice day, or in a room other than the cafeteria. This does involve packing the lunch, which you can do the night before. The easy part is that you already know the pattern. A piece of fruit, milk, and a vegetable (raw carrots?). Then add a sandwich or leftovers.

If your frantic schedule continues through the evening and keeps you from having a pleasant dinner, that's a shame. Similarly, if you arrive home for dinner but are so hungry that you've already eaten in the car, or you grab some snack food as soon as you walk in the door, thereby "spoiling your dinner" (there's that no-no again), you're missing out on one of life's great pleasures.

PATTERN: NIGHT WORK

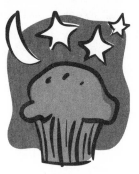

WORKING THROUGH THE NIGHT is hazardous to your health if you don't have the opportunity to eat regular meals. The tempting baked goods and other treats your co-workers bring in don't help, either. Your colleagues and your friends want to help you with this difficult shift by feeding you.

Let's say you work in a hospital. The cafeteria is closed in the middle of the night, or it has a limited selection: pre-wrapped sandwiches and snack food. Maybe, just maybe, a speckled apple or an over-ripe

THE HEALTHY WEIGH, 1890 VERSION: Some things never change: "The hurry and unrest of contemporary life do not conduce the appreciation of fine cooking. . . ." Arthur Child, "Delicate Feasting."

banana. Probably closed, though. Most likely you'll be hitting the vending machines, with all the chips and cookies and sodas your little heart desires. See those empty compartments? That's where the fruit should be.

Let's say you are protecting our streets at night. The men in blue. The women in blue. Are you protecting the people who work in all-night doughnut shops by taking your break there? It can be a social break, too, since you see the same people night after night. But doughnut shops don't offer much in the way of food selection, and aren't known for what you'd call "full meals." Lucky for you if you take your break in a 24-hour diner.

Now let's say you are a factory worker on swing shift. You have no control over the time of your meals, which change according to your work schedule. (We saw a billboard in Atlanta that said, "Stomachs can't tell time. 24 hours — Denny's." Your job is to teach your stomach to tell time.) Maybe you can't relate to mealtimes because you eat whenever you can, which bears no relation to when the rest of your town eats. Still, we'll bet that you do have three meals. It's just that you probably have three dinners.

So you'll want to form new meal patterns, which are, ironically, the old three meals a day: breakfast, lunch, and dinner. One of the meals is breakfast, and you use breakfast foods for that. Another meal is lunch, and … you know the rest. The point is that your three meals *cannot*, repeat *cannot* all be dinner. (By the way, they can't all be snacks, either, an eating trap when you're hungry and tired. Night workers find snacking the easiest way to eat, but it's far, far from the best.)

The ball's in your court now. You have to plan to get these three meals into your day, albeit a very different kind of day. Of course these meals have to be healthy ones. This is more difficult when you are working through the night, because your options are extremely limited, and your chances of finding fruits, vegetables, low-fat dairy, and whole grains are slim to none. If you don't want to bring food from home, ask your favorite restaurant manager to have these things available. You can start a whole campaign, maybe get people to sign a petition. Suddenly the newspapers will get hold of it and do a story! Your local television station will interview you! You'll be famous! And all because you wanted a dish of cut-up fruit, some

THE HEALTHY WEIGH: If you aren't sleeping well, night shift or no, talk to your doctor. Tiredness takes its toll. Besides, it makes losing weight a difficult proposition.

fresh spinach, a glass of low-fat milk, and a little brown rice.

Do you remember "Life With Fruit" from The Best Foods on Earth chapter? Here it is again, but rewritten and re-titled, just for you.

LIFE WITH MEALS

Breakfast in the night?
Whole wheat roll will make it right.
Have milk and apple, too,
It's a simple thing to do.

Please, don't forget your juice.
(Do we sound like Dr. Seuss?)
Fruit at breakfast leads the way –
In your new meal pattern day.

For lunch? Do salads, please,
They are diner specialties.
Would they add some fruit as well?
Plus a glass of milk? That's swell!

With dinner — veggies (green),
They're the best you've ever seen.
For dessert — some cut-up fruit.
Easy living — what a hoot!

You'll probably want an entree at lunch, certainly at dinner. Even though we didn't memorialize the main course of the meal in rhyme, low fat is still the way to go. Check out the section called "'DASH' Dining for Dummies" a little farther along.

PATTERN: BEHIND THE SCENES

CONVINCED THAT YOU HAVE TO have three meals a day? Making sure you eat them is a challenge. It was a lot easier when Mom did all the cooking. She also did a lot behind the scenes, probably while you were at school. She made out her shopping list, went to the grocery store, bought the fruits and vegetables and milk and everything else on her list, took it all home and put it away, one of the more thankless tasks. Unless she's still doing that, you're going to have to figure out how Mom did it. We can pull the curtain and look behind the scenes to see what Mom's magic was all about.

Well, like the Wizard of Oz, it turns out that Mom's "magic" wasn't magic at all. It was organization. That's what we see when we look behind the curtain, and that's what we'll look at now. Mom knew how to make the most of her trips to the grocery store.

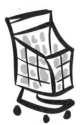

Pattern: Shopping

SOME PEOPLE ENJOY SHOPPING and some don't. Whether you like it or not, you have to go to the store. We think of what Willie Sutton said when someone asked him why he robbed banks: "That's where the money is." Well, the reason you have to go to the supermarket is because that's where the food is. Even if someone volunteers to do your shopping for you, it won't do you any good if you haven't explored the territory and really seen what's there. There is territory to explore, too, in the new-and-improved food stores, which have grown to such a size that some of them deserve to have their own zip codes. They are super-supermarkets. Fortunately they are stocked with all sorts of surprises. Unfortunately they really could use shuttle service to get you from one end to the other. And it wouldn't hurt them to give you a map.

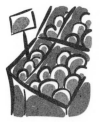

Pattern: Learning the Ropes

THE NEXT TIME YOU GO FOOD SHOPPING, think of it as a brand new experience. Break your routine and explore the aisles. This is a themed shopping expedition, one that has you looking for new fruits and vegetables to try. You might discover a new taste treat — red pepper spread, for instance. You just might find yourself part of a new trend.

For those in the market for variety, there are many, many vegetables to choose from, and they don't go out of season, either. Bell peppers, for instance, can be found in more than just traditional Christmas colors — yellow, purple, and deep orange. Mushrooms are not just those that look like little drawings in children's stories. There are also shiitake (tiny parasols), huge Portobello (beach umbrellas), and enoki (large toothpicks with tiny hats) to name just a few.

Be sure to visit the aisles that will increase the likelihood that you will fill your cart with fruits, vegetables, whole grains, and low-fat dairy. We're always on the lookout for interestingly packaged vegetables we might never have seen before, and fruits from all around the world.

LET'S HEAR IT FOR VARIETY

"Temperate" fruits don't have a temper,
They come from the temperate zone.
Citrus fruits are always juicy,
They grow where the sun has shown.
Tropical fruits like the hot, hot weather,
Berries think it's better cool.
Melons grow where it's not too sultry
Melons are nobody's fool.
Cut up fruit and call it a "cocktail,"
Pretty and hard to beat.
Juices are great — no need to chew 'em!
It's fruit! It's a super treat!

Then there are glass jars filled with fruits and vegetables, frequently unusual ones, and it's nice to see what you're getting. There are wonderful canned foods as well. Check out the greens that are packed in there. Collard greens, beet greens, kale — well worth trying. Don't forget about beets, recipe-ready diced tomatoes, and pineapple "tidbits."

Move on to frozen foods and see what's new and different there. Frozen vegetables have gone far beyond peas and carrots to include such items as asparagus, artichoke hearts, and snow peas. Even if you've never been too crazy about frozen vegetables, you might want to try them. You will discover frozen pearl onions and — a very big hit — frozen chopped onions, which really should be called "No Tears." Dried apricots and prunes are on the shelf, but so are "Goldens and Cherries," "Fruit Bits," and "Tropical Medley," all tiny delights by Sun-Maid.

As for grains — besides the obvious bread and cereal aisles, explore the aisle where whole grains are found. Try a different brand or a different type of rice, maybe wild rice or brown rice. (Uncle Ben's Brown Rice makes a nice transition, being less heavy than other brown rices. Takes less time to cook than they do, too.). Have you ever tried barley? Now's your chance. Try a new taste treat, like dried sweet corn. By the way — store the opened package of whole grains in a zip-lock bag, so that it will last longer.

Go to several different food markets in your area, and find the one you feel most comfortable wandering around in, one that has the selection best suited to your needs. Maybe you've never been in one of these places before, but they do exist. If you enjoy (or, at the very least, don't mind) being in your food store, life will improve immeasurably.

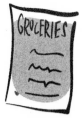

Pattern:
Healthy Hoarding

EVERYTHING REQUIRES PLANNING. Think of prison escapes. Well, the same goes for grocery shopping, and you won't need a blunt instrument, either. You are working behind the scenes now, putting together a secret stash of healthy foods that won't spoil, that stand ready for duty when fresh versions are missing in action. This was part of Mom's organization, and you can do likewise. All you need is shelf and freezer space, and the determination to use and replace these items as needed.

Why are you doing this? Because keeping good, healthy foods around increases your chances of eating them. So here is a checklist for what you need in the house. This is not your shopping list, because only you know what you are making for dinner. Rather it is "healthy hoarding."

- Dried fruits
- Canned fruits ("lite," in juice rather than syrup)
- Fruit juice
- Canned vegetables, no salt added
- Canned tomatoes (ditto)
- Spaghetti sauce (ditto)
- Canned soups, low sodium (vegetable, lentil, split pea)
- Frozen vegetables
- Nonfat dry milk
- Oatmeal and other whole grain cereals
- Brown rice
- whole grain pastas
- Microwave popcorn, low fat
- Dried beans, legumes, lentils
- Canned salmon and canned tuna packed in water
- Frozen fish (not breaded)
- Chicken breasts, lean cuts of beef (to be frozen)
- Vinegar, olive oil, canola oil, cooking spray
- Salad dressings
- Mustard, ketchup

THE HEALTHY WEIGH: Healthy hoarding does not include a super-size package of snack food. And — the more snack foods you have in your house, the harder it will be to lose weight.

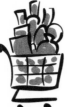

Pattern: Filling the Shopping Cart

IT'S TIME FOR A WEEKLY SHOPPING TRIP, and you'll begin by doing your "healthy hoarding." Next week, all you'll have to do is replenish your stash.

You are going to need lots of fruits and vegetables, a WHOLE lot, because you're buying a week's worth. We've already talked about how you are going to get those "High Five! Try Five!" (five fruits, five vegetables) and "Hi Ho, the Dairy-o" (low fat, naturally) into your day, but how are you going to get them into your house? How are you going to get this food in hand so you can have it on hand? Which you have to do, because, as we've said before, your best shot at really eating all those fruits and vegetables and drinking that juice is to make sure they are, in fact, in the house.

You may never have thought to buy in bulk before, but remember, you're stocking up, and you'll need plenty to see you through the week. Go for the bags of apples, oranges, and potatoes. While you're at it, take a stroll around the produce section and see what might look good in your salad. Buy a featured fruit, maybe pears. How do you know when they're ripe? We know of a young man who asked another shopper, also buying the unripe pears that were for sale, how to tell when they were ripe. She explained that he should put the pears on the window sill for a few days, and that he should squeeze them from time to time to test their ripeness. He went up to her in the checkout line and handed her his telephone number. He hoped, he said, she'd call him when her pears were ripe.

The fruit you buy doesn't all have to be fresh, as should, by now, be obvious. It might be canned, it might be dried — both handy as back-up when your bananas turn black. (By the way — you can use that black banana in a FAST AND FRUITY BREAKFAST shake — see p. 198) By using them, you'll wind up with more variety and less spoilage. Go up and down the aisles and get the canned and frozen fruits (don't forget juice) and the vegetables that you staked out on your last expedition. Get the whole grains and dairy, too

Keep an eye on your shopping cart. Does it appear to be filling with mostly fruits and vegetables, maybe some bread, cereals, and other grains? How about low-fat dairy? That's the idea.

When you get everything home and are putting it away, see what fruits need further ripening, so that you can leave those on the windowsill rather than put them right into the refrigerator. Bananas are a special case, as the old jingle says. They come from the "tropical Equator," and "so you must never put [them] in the refrigerator!" Like bananas, many fruits and vegetables have their ripening idiosyncrasies, so be like the pear-buying guy in the supermarket and ask someone.

The fresh fruits and vegetables that you are putting into the refrigerator should not be pushed to the back. Out of sight is out of mind, not a good thing here. Make sure you see them — and eat them. We know a woman who puts three pieces of fruit out on the counter every morning, and makes sure she has eaten them by the time she goes to bed. You could do the same. Or you could take that fruit to work, display it on your desk, and eat it with pride. Start a trend — fruit has the distinct edge when it comes to portability.

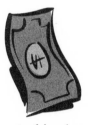

Pattern: Spending Money

ALL OF THIS NEW SHOPPING may call for a shift in mindset, because you're shifting the way you spend your money — less on soda, snacks, and meats, and more on fruits, vegetables, low-fat dairy, and whole grains. What you are buying is health. Why does the cost of buying pre-washed lettuce prevent you from putting it into your shopping cart, but not the cost of an extra-large bag of chips, for example? Forgive the expression, but you're comparing apples and oranges. Certainly the bag of chips is bigger ("Super Size" says the 20-ounce bag), and you may feel that you are getting more for your money, but what is it you are buying? More important, what is it you are eating? In the case of chips versus pre-washed lettuce, you are choosing to spend your money on a whole lot of snack food rather than on a convenient way to eat vegetables. The chips path is seductive, though, and along the way you'll find occasional money-saving enticements in the form of coupons ("Buy 2! Save $1 now!"), which means you throw them into your cart even faster than usual. There is virtually no chance that you'll go back and buy that bag of pre-washed lettuce, is there? You figure that by the time you've eaten half the chips on the way home, you won't have any room left for vegetables anyway, so why buy them? Well, to get yourself healthier, for one thing.

THE HEALTHY WEIGH: Have a week's worth of fruits and vegetables in your house: dried, canned, fresh, or frozen.

It's no more expensive to build your meals around plenty of fruits and vegetables than it is to build around anything else. The DASH study used data compiled by government surveys, and determined that the amount of money necessary to follow the DASH diet falls within the budget of average Americans. Money is not the issue, and should not stand between you and fruits and vegetables.

So save some of that grocery money for fruits, vegetables, low-fat dairy, and whole grains. It will go farther if you find a produce market, farm market, or food co-op. You may have to go a little out of your way, but it's worth it.

If you are a smoker and are complaining that fruits and vegetables cost too much, we don't want to hear it. Not with the current price of a carton of cigarettes.

PATTERN: EQUIPMENT

CONSIDER BUYING A FEW THINGS that will make life easier for your future in the kitchen. A new pattern. These handy-dandy pieces of equipment will further increase the likelihood that you'll eat lots of fruits and vegetables. You may have thought of these "gadgets" as superfluous, but think again. They are really helpful.

Plastic roll-up cutting board — you'll be chopping a lot of vegetables, and this cutting board beats your heavy, wooden one in a number of ways. The plastic one (very thin and flat) goes in the dishwasher and stores easily. It lets you carry the chopped vegetables to a pot, bowl, or whatever, and then bend it to form a kind of spout, allowing you to pour the vegetables into the container rather than onto the floor.

Good can opener — are you avoiding opening canned fruit because your hand hurts when you use your can opener? Try a new can opener. Modern ones are a big improvement over their ancestors. The new ones are easy to turn, easy to hold. Good looking, too.

Microwave dish with lid — you'll be microwaving a lot of vegetables. Do you have a history of destroying plastic containers by putting them in the microwave? Help is on the way. Time to move up in the world to a special dish that can withstand the heat.

Nice, large salad bowl — is the size of your salad dictated by the size of the bowl you have in the house? Do you make a mess tossing your salad because the bowl is too small? Your new purchase will encourage you to make more salad and take more salad. When you use a smaller bowl, it looks like there's not enough, so people won't take much, even if there's more in the kitchen and you were planning to refill.

Kitchen scissors — maybe you've never thought a pair of scissors belonged in the kitchen, but it's better than teeth for opening packages. Invaluable for cutting up chives, sundried tomatoes, and loads of other things. Little things. Gets those fat globules off the chicken, too.

Rubber garlic tube — invaluable for users of fresh garlic. Just put a couple of cloves into the tube, roll it around with the palm of your hand, and you'll find the garlic skin comes off easily. Amazing! A word of caution — this is fun, and you have to be careful not to over-do it, or you'll wind up with a lot more peeled garlic than you need.

Garlic press — avoiding fresh garlic because you don't want to peel and chop? Drop a clove in the press and squeeze — or buy a jar of ready-chopped garlic.

Apple peeler, corer — this gets the "Authors' Choice" award. Just the look is entertaining, and it certainly has the flavor of history. As you just saw in the Connection, it's even listed as one of the 93 "essential" kitchen items for the 1880 cook. If you want to witness the magic of having an apple cored, peeled, and sliced, this is for you. Even if you have no plans to make applesauce, get one anyway. The grandkids will love it.

"Blender on a Stick" — with this "immersion blender," you can throw some cut-up vegetables and potatoes into a pot, cook them for awhile, and purée them with this little wonder. And you can do it right in the pot! Voilà — soup! Creamy and delicious, without the cream. A vast improvement over dumping the hot liquid into a food processor, where the heat creates suction that makes the top almost impossible to get off — but that's another story.

PATTERN: "DASH" DINING FOR DUMMIES

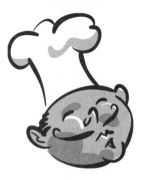

NOW THAT YOU KNOW HOW to do the shopping and you have the equipment, you just have to decide whether or not you want to do the cooking. If not, you can hire a personal chef, an individual who loves to cook and will cater to your tastes and preferences. This person will make specially designed meals for you, either in your own kitchen or not. The food can be delivered to your house, already prepared. In fact, home-delivered meals are a growth industry. Or you can stop and pick up ready-made meals at the grocery store or your favorite restaurant. Okay, dinner's ready.

If you are going to be cooking, you need a treasure trove of entree recipes, your keys to easy dinner making. You'll want variety in these recipes: chicken, turkey, beef, pork, fish, seafood, vegetarian. Clearly, if you have food allergies, food preferences, religious or cultural issues, you might have to eliminate some. In any event, use these recipes over and over again. No surprises. They may be old family favorites, or ones you clipped from the newspaper, or saw on a television cooking show. As long as they're low fat , which may require adaptation, and they work for you, that's all that matters.

Tired of your recipes? Try the "14-Day Meal Plan With Meal Appeal" later in this book. Let us do the planning. Don't make extra work for yourself. Just use these recipes on a regular basis. There's something to be said for repetition. If the food tastes good, people won't mind that a given dinner appears from time to time. They may even look forward to it.

Now you need to have a grocery list that includes all the ingredients from those recipes. Thanks to your healthy hoarding, you'll discover that you already have some of these ingredients in the house, and the rest you're about to go and buy. Definitely make that list. You may think you'll remember everything, the way you still remember the names of all your first-grade classmates. You have all the best intentions, but then you run into a friend in the supermarket, chat for awhile, and by the time you get to the parking lot you realize you are missing key ingredients for tonight's dinner. Count yourself lucky. At least you can go back inside and buy what you need. You might have found yourself in front of the stove at dinnertime before the thought occurred to you.

DASH Dining for Dummies includes a night out at least once a week, plus a night or two of take-out (to be discussed shortly). Your organizing includes delegating tasks, training other members of the household so that they, too, are a part of this event called "making dinner." You might even delegate the entire dinner, not washing your hands of it, but forming a partnership in the dinner production, which includes the whole deal — list-making, grocery shopping, and, of course, cooking. We know a woman who has three teenagers, and each cooks one night every week. You never know!

PATTERN: CREATING AMBIANCE
Basic

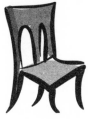

YOU'RE ASSUMING CANDLELIGHT, linen table-cloths, and numerous courses, aren't you? Well, we're here to present a more basic approach to ambiance, one that involves a table and chairs. Simple but nice. Sitting down is good, even key. If you stand up to eat, that's what you are doing. Eating. You have to be sitting down to have it qualify as "dinner."

It's nice when the house smells good, and you don't have to pre-pare a lot of courses to have the house smell good, either. You can even pretend cook. If you sauté some onions, people will think things are happening at dinner time. This will give you a chance to figure out what in the world to make for dinner — which may or may not have anything to do with onions. For a dessert smell, put some grapes in the oven to bake slowly (see recipe for Granny Grapes, p. 162)

Dinnertime is a good time, worth being awake for. If dinnertime competes with bedtime, either you're going to bed too early or you're eating too late. Do some planning to avoid severe overlap. Make time for these two important events in your day and give them their due.

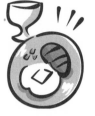

Advanced

YOU CAN MAKE FOOD LOOK BEAUTIFUL, maybe use a pretty stemmed glass for some fruit, because, if you think about it, you'll realize *you eat first with your eyes*. Have different colors on your plate (deep green asparagus, golden sweet potato). Then when you are sitting down to a good meal, you'll have visual pleasure as well. Good smells will fill the house, and you can focus on other things — conversation, for instance. Companionship. Or, if you're alone, maybe a good book keeps you quiet company, or a cross-word puzzle. Put on some music, or the news. Sit a bit and appreciate the food, appreciate the evening, relax. This is a special time of the day, and you deserve to enjoy it.

PATTERN: COMPANY COMING

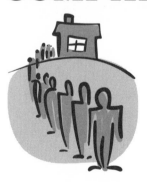

THE WAY YOU LEARN a new pattern is to repeat it over and over again. Then you're ready to go public, and here's a great way to do just that. If things go well, which they will, you'll be on your way to developing an enviable reputation for serving lots of delicious fruits and vegetables. The brunch that follows is a golden opportunity to show off how easy it is to work them into your eating day, and how pleasurable it can be to eat them. In this wonderful, colorful meal, you will count EIGHT different fruits and vegetables, plus a little low-fat dairy and whole grain. It is the culmination of all the new patterns you have put in place. Congratulations! You have a right to be proud.

"DASH OF PRIDE" BRUNCH
YIN AND YANG SOUP (see recipe, page 191)
MASHED POTATOES, SWEET POTATOES, CARROTS (see recipe,
page 186)
ROASTED RED BEET SALAD (see recipe, page 184)
Entrée of your choice
(may we suggest broiled salmon or grilled chicken breast)
Whole- or multi-grain bread or rolls
GORGEOUS FRUIT CUSTARD (see recipe, page 199)

PATTERN: RESTAURANTS

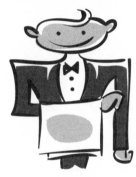

REMEMBER THE OLD BLUE PLATE SPE-CIAL? Three compartments, the biggest one of which had meat, and the two smaller ones had a greenish vegetable in one and mashed potatoes in the other? Now update it! Fill 1/2 your plate with vegetables, 1/4 with whole grains, and 1/4 with meat, poultry, beans, whatever. It's the new, improved blue plate special. (Word of this has yet to reach restaurants, by the way.)

Restaurants are part of life. If you go often, it's a convenience, not a big treat, so you'll want to use the "blue plate special" method. One thing is sure — you are going to get a great big serving of meat or poultry or fish. Restaurants know that you expect to "get your money's worth," which translates into enormous portions guaranteed to make sure you gain weight. So decide right now, before you even leave the house, that you are going to take half of your meat home, which means you'll get to enjoy it twice as often. Double your pleasure.

When you order your I-know-I'm-taking-half-of-this-home dinner, think "no cream, no cheese, no butter" to keep the fat down. Yours too. Talk to the server and see how dishes are prepared. We had an experience when we ordered baked tilapia (a delicious white fish) that was served on a bed of rice. Silly us. We neglected to ask if there

THE HEALTHY WEIGH: If you're trying to lose weight, eat out no more than three meals per week.

would be melted cheese between the rice and the fish! You never know, so you just have to say, "Please — no cream, no cheese, no butter."

You still have half the blue plate special to fill, so ask about vegetables. Make sure to ask for extras. Is there a "vegetable of the day"? Does the table next to yours feature something on a beautiful bed of asparagus? See if you can have that with your order. If you fail in all of the above attempts to get extra vegetables, try for vegetable soup. Salad, absolutely. Every restaurant offers it.

Think fruit for dessert. Unfortunately it's the fashion these days to come around with a dessert tray — or a dessert CART — that's loaded with all kinds of beautiful rich, creamy, high-fat desserts. Somebody apparently figured out that if you actually see and smell the chocolate nut buttercream torte you're much more likely to order it than if you just read about it on the menu. But be creative. You can mix and match. Maybe they have a cheesecake with a raspberry sauce. And maybe you remember there was a fresh fruit appetizer. Ask if you might have the raspberry sauce over the fresh fruit. Maybe they have a sorbet they can put on top of that. You have a wonderful, delicious, fruitful dessert.

Sometimes when you eat out, you also eat *up* — on an airplane. Whatever you do, when you leave home, don't go hungry. When you're hungry, your goal is simply to fill your stomach and you'll grab anything handy. Only later do you reconsider, and lament, what you had to eat. When you are traveling, you need something to tide you over until you get some real food. Take a couple of bagels as well as apples and bananas for the ride. Chances are that it will be a long time until beverage service, and you will have a good, filling, not particularly messy snack to munch on. For a longer flight, you can find out in advance if your flight offers meals (less and less likely) when you book your reservation. If it does, call ahead and order a fresh fruit plate. Fruit with every meal — and every flight. Otherwise take food with you. Remember: fruit, vegetable, low-fat dairy, and whole grains. But let's get back to earth.

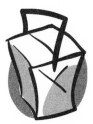

Pattern: Take-Out

CALL IT TAKE-OUT, TAKE-IN, OR TAKE-AWAY as they do in England, somebody else cooked it, and you bought it and took it home. Maybe it's Chinese food, maybe pizza, maybe subs/hoagies/grinders. These all have something in common, which is that they are high in fat. This automatically makes them "special occasion" fare. Ironic, huh? Here you are, buying pretty inexpensive, readily available food, which may have been your dinner every night since you can remember, and now it's a "birthdays only" thing. But if you still want these foods every day, one possibility is low-fat variations. For Chinese, choose steamed vegetables with chicken or shrimp. For pizza, order extra vegetables instead of the usual (high in fat) pepperoni or sausage. While you're at it, ask for half the cheese. In fact, many places now make delicious no-cheese pizzas. Finally, find a pizza place that also has salad. Then buy it.

As for subs/hoagies/grinders, go for turkey (or ham or beef) with lots of vegetables and Italian dressing on the side. If you see a salad-type, such as tuna salad, run the other way. This is NOT the kind of salad we keep talking about. As for mayonnaise — they'll be very generous in their use of this high-fat spread, so don't use it unless this is a special occasion. If they are advertising two-foot hoagies, consider that 4 inches is about right, so you're looking at enough for a family of six.

There are other places to get take out, places where you might find low-fat food — restaurants. Lots of restaurants love you if you order by phone and pick up the food to go. It's free money for them, since they don't have to supply a server, table linens, and so on, they don't have to wash your dishes, and, best of all from their point of view, you will not be taking up a table. Collect menus and familiarize yourself with low-fat choices. Think vegetables. They may have a good selection of "sides." Remember to double your pleasure, since the meat/poultry/fish will serve you tonight and again tomorrow night if you play your cards right.

Supermarkets have whole sections of prepared foods, and they often come already doled out in microwaveable containers. Or you can have someone behind the counter put together a plate for you. Same deal, though — make sure you're getting low fat and plenty of vegetables.

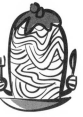

"All You Can Eat" Places

THE THING IS, you take it as a challenge: "I'll show them how much I can eat!" and then you go to it. But keep in mind that when you eat, the idea is to use a fork, not a forklift. You can't blame your monstrous serving size on the restaurant, because you serve yourself. Our view of these places is best summed up in the following:

A VIRGINIA REEL FOR REAL PEOPLE
"All you can eat," says the restaurant sign.
"C'mon in, it's the place to dine!
"Step right up, get your money's worth!
"Best darn food anywhere on earth!"
But if you're smart, you'll drive on by,
Don't even think about it, my-oh-my!
Swing your partner, do-si-do,
Now you find another place to go!
Hey, everybody, tall and short!
EATING IS NOT A COMPETITIVE SPORT!

PATTERN: GET A GRIP

AS A CULTURE WE have always appreciated bigger than life, and now everybody is bigger than life. "Get a grip" refers to the fact that you can pretty much see how big your portions should be by using your hands as a measure. Kind of a rule of thumb. Get it? For healthy eating and Nutrition Facts, you hear a lot about measuring. You don't have to carry around measuring cups and spoons and a scale. Look at these pictures:

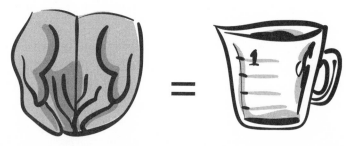

PATTERN: FAMILIES

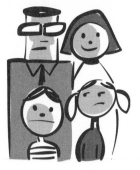

WHAT STAGE ARE YOU IN? If you have young children around, you have a fair amount of influence over what they eat. It is your responsibility to make sure they are getting all the healthy foods they need, and you know what they are, because they are the same for you. You are the gatekeeper — buying these foods, making them available, having them conveniently located in the refrigerator and on the counter, serving them at meals, and eating them yourself. You create an atmosphere that will encourage, if not insure, healthy eating in your house. You are probably giving them some choices, not too many, because it's confusing. We love the story (true) of the woman who was on the phone activating her Discover card. She gave some information and was put on hold, at which point her three-year-old son came in, looking for a snack. The woman offered carrots, crackers, pretzels, cereal, juice box, raisins. The Discover woman came back on and said, "Okay, your card is activated. And you're giving him way too many choices."

Obviously, the older the children, the less your influence. And if they are adults, you may have no influence at all — or, ironically, much more than you realize. You do what you do, you have a wonderful, healthy lifestyle, and maybe, just maybe, some of it will rub off. If people are paying attention to you, it's not for fashion trends (that's for sure), not for hair styles (obviously), but if you're really paying attention to food, they'll notice. One way they'll know you are paying attention is that they see you choosing a smaller size drink at a fast food restaurant, knowing the Big Gulp isn't the best choice.

The family pattern starts with you when you embrace your own healthy eating lifestyle. Then you set up a structure so that others follow your lead. That's about all you can do.

MOM KNEW BEST
"An apple a day
Keeps the doctor away" —
And what made Popeye strong?

THE HEALTHY WEIGH: Impress your family! Choose smaller sizes at fast food places.

He finished his spinach
With joy undiminished —
We've known it all along.

"Now drink your milk!
It's smooth as silk!"
We heard our mothers say.

"So drink it down
Without a frown,
And do it every day."

Well, Mom knew best
We can attest.
This makes an ideal diet.

Eat veggies, fruit,
Drink milk, to boot,
Be healthy — why not try it?

PATTERN: EXERCISE

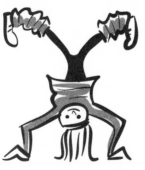

JUST BECAUSE THIS BOOK has no separate chapter entitled "Exercise! Do It or Rue It!" doesn't mean you get a pass on exercising. Developing a pattern for exercise is an important part of your new, healthy lifestyle. You have to move every day, in some way, shape, or form. This need not be a traditional spandex workout. You just want to do something that will make your heart beat faster and make you breathe harder, which will, in turn, get more oxygen into you.

Your workout can be as simple as brisk walking. It may help to think of this as "having someplace to go." The workout can be traditional — biking, hiking, playing sports — or nontraditional — dancing or rowing or vigorous orchestra-leading. You just have to do it, so if there's no lake or orchestra nearby, find something else you enjoy doing. That's the key — enjoyment. If you like what you're doing, you automatically increase the likelihood that you'll do it.

How much exercise do you need? In a word, *more*. More than you are getting now. Let's talk minutes. Since 1996, the recommendation has been at least 30 minutes of "moderate activity" on most days. Now the bar has been raised. New government guidelines (a 1,000-page report, if you must know) include those for exercise, and it all boils down to this (are you sitting down?): *at least one hour of exercise every day in order to maintain health and normal weight.* These are the guidelines, but that's all they are — guidelines. One hour is the gold standard, and a goal, but don't give it all up because it seems overwhelming. You can only do what you can do.

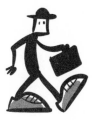

You and Your Pedometer

"WAIT A MINUTE," we hear you protest. "I don't have to exercise, because I move around a lot at work." Well, let's see what that really means. Get yourself a pedometer, a small, inexpensive, clip-on gizmo that, when properly set, counts the steps you take and prominently displays the information. Just hook it on your waistband, and away you go. Maybe. In fact, that's what you're about to find out, because your pedometer will keep track of the number of steps you take, the steps of everyday life, not just those you take when exercising. These include walking around the supermarket, playing with your children or grandchildren, cleaning the house, and so on.

You just may find you don't move around as much as you think you do. This is understandable. It's a toxic exercise environment, and everything is conspiring to keep you from being active. You have wheels on your chair that will scoot you around your work area. You can e-mail an office-mate who sits twenty feet away rather than walk over for an in-person visit. You have a cell phone for personal calls, so you don't have to go down the hall to the pay phone. You can fax directly from your computer rather than walk to the fax machine. Work stations have been specifically designed to minimize steps. While this maximizes efficiency, it minimizes your opportuni-

THE HEALTHY WEIGH: Exercise more. Just do the best you can.

ty to boost the numbers on your pedometer.

So you can use your pedometer in two ways. First, you can keep track of the steps you take; second, you can notice when the numbers are low, your signal that it's time to get up and move around. You might like to know that studies show simply wearing a pedometer makes people take more steps. Very sedentary people take 3,000 steps a day. Same for people with knee problems, or serious disease. People who are normal weight are likely to take about 10,000 steps each day. In fact, walking 10,000 steps a day can lower blood pressure and lower your cholesterol. All you need are feet and a sidewalk.

One of us wore a pedometer and discovered that, while sitting at work, she, too, took only about 3,000 steps a day. When she added an early-morning walk, she took about 7,000 steps. When she added a visit with her grandchildren — wow! 14,000 steps! That's what you get for having young grandchildren who want to be carried everywhere.

THE HEALTHY WEIGH:
Take 10,000 steps a day.

IN A NUTSHELL:
Start today! Do each of the following:
- Eat three meals — breakfast, lunch, and dinner.
- Buy a new grain and make it for dinner.
- If you go to a restaurant, order an extra vegetable — and have fruit for dessert.
- Do more exercise today than you did yesterday.

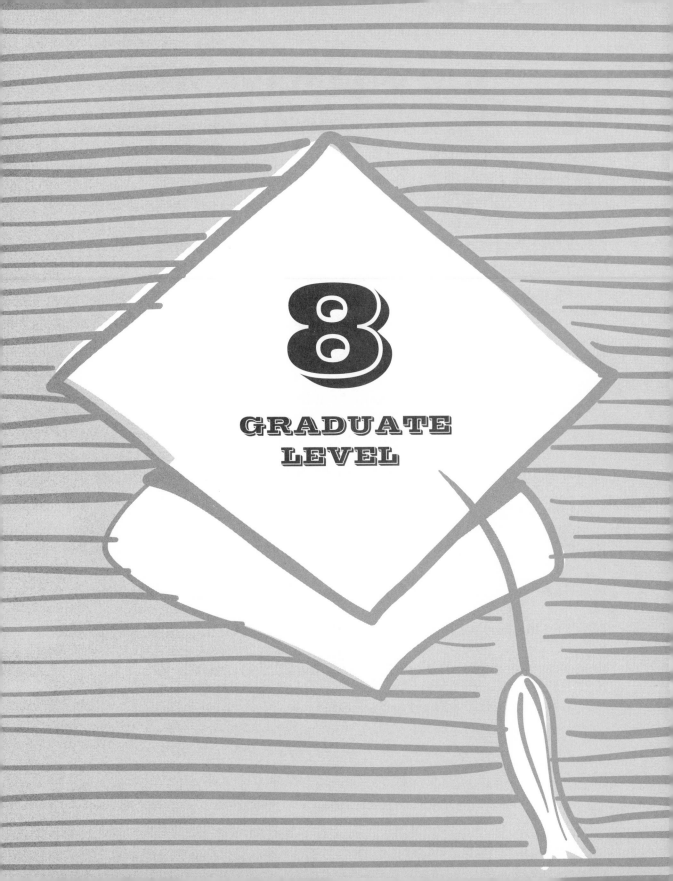

8

GRADUATE
LEVEL

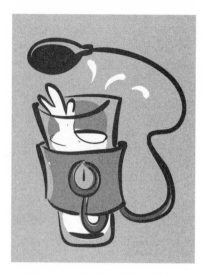

THE DASH DIET

AS YOU KNOW, everything in this book has been based on DASH, a major study by the National Institutes of Health. The goal was to see if it lowered blood pressure, and it did. People ate lots of fruits, vegetables, and low-fat dairy. These three foods lowered blood pressure. Our view throughout *The Best Diet On Earth* has been to take this and make it larger, since, as we noted in the Introduction, the researchers themselves called it "the diet for all diseases." In addition to lowering blood pressure, researchers believe that the Dash diet will also lower the risk of heart disease, diabetes, and cancer. Think about it, one diet to prevent the Big Four diseases, the Chronic Ones. ★ Little by little, we are testing DASH. As you will see later in the Graduate Level, the DASH diet is indeed lowering markers for heart disease. All indications are that time will prove the researchers right. But before we examine these markers, let's look at a few "odds and ends" related to the DASH diet, namely, sodium and sweets.

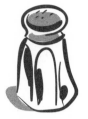

Sodium

"HOW ABOUT SODIUM?" you ask. "I thought lowering sodium was what lowered blood pressure." In fact, the DASH diet was not particularly low in sodium, although it wasn't high, either. The foods were all naturally low in sodium (fruits, vegetables, low-fat dairy, and whole grains). Participants did not, however, have any salty snacks. For their listening pleasure, they were given tiny little packets of salt to add to their food, if they wanted. Sprinkling a small amount of salt on top of the food after cooking gives it a salty taste, with less salt than if it was mixed in. It fools your palate. "Surface salting," this is called. (Who knew there was a term for these things?)

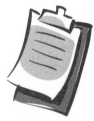

Sodium and Another DASH Study

RESEARCHERS ARE NEVER SATISFIED, and this was no exception. They published another study, one that looked at the effects of the DASH-diet-plus-sodium-reduction on blood pressure. There were three groups. The first was assigned a sodium intake based on the original DASH diet. The second had less sodium, because researchers believed that they could get blood pressure lower than they did with the original diet. And they could, making it a reasonable option for real people who want to take DASH one step further ("DASH-Sodium") to lower their blood pressure. Then — well, there was the third group, and they had *half the amount of the second group!* Yes, their blood pressure was somewhat lower than the second group's, but what can we say about their diet? Basically it was so low in sodium that they couldn't swim in the ocean.

As researchers had thought, less sodium does indeed mean further reduction in blood pressure. But there is the lingering question: How long can people realistically stay on a very, very low sodium diet? Who knows? It's a question for the ages.

Meanwhile, if we were hat wearers, we would take off our hats to the DASH researchers. They have shown that The Best Foods on Earth are the basis of a wonderful, healthy diet, and for that, we thank them.

THE HEALTHY WEIGH:
Use less salt.

Sodium and You

SO — HERE YOU ARE, trying to live the DASH way, and one way to do that is cut down on sodium. Here are some tips.

☞ Eat foods in their original form (fruits, vegetables, and whole grains) which are naturally low in sodium, as are fresh meats.

☞ For packaged foods, use Nutrition Facts, and stay with "less than 5% Daily Value" for sodium. By the way, you won't be seeing that on a salty snack label any time soon, and there aren't many processed foods like lunch meats, ham, bacon, etc. that qualify, either. (To repeat, you can be sure there were no salty snacks in the DASH study.)

☞ Fill your salt shaker with pepper.

☞ When cooking or baking, look for recipes that don't use baking soda or baking powder, both of which are really high in sodium.

☞ Be on the lookout for sodium in commonly used food flavorings and condiments, like soy sauce, packaged seasoning mixes, and so on. Obviously, garlic salt and onion salt are just what they say they are — salt.

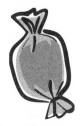

DASH and Sweets

IF YOU HAVE A SWEET TOOTH, the DASH diet will present something of a challenge. First of all, participants had only *five servings per week.* If you'll recall, there are seven days in a week, not five, which means that two sweet-less days are left hanging. Then, too, what is considered a serving is pretty small. Some examples: 1/2 cup low-fat or fat-free frozen yogurt;1 tablespoon of sugar; 1 tablespoon of jelly or jam; 8 ounces lemonade or fruit punch (sweetened with sugar, obviously). This means that if you put some jam or your toast in the morning, that's it. Your sweet for the day. Certainly the way to eat if you want to lose weight.

A real problem with eating a lot of sweets is that you have neither the opportunity nor the inclination to eat the good stuff, which is what the DASH diet is all about. But if the limit on sweets sounds difficult for you, not to worry. Remember — any step, no matter how

THE HEALTHY WEIGH:

Make whole grains your new "sweets."

small, is a step in the right direction. We admire you enormously for making the effort.

HEALTH MARKERS

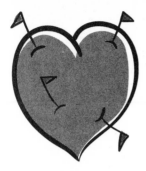

THERE IS A RELATIONSHIP between heart health and diet. We can actually look at markers in your blood to tell us how healthy you are. What are these markers?

LDL Cholesterol

THIS MARKER HAS A FAMILIAR RING: cholesterol. You have heard about it for a long time. You may know that your body manufactures it. You may not know that cholesterol travels in your blood in different guises: LDL, HDL and VLDL. Because one of these guises can cause heart disease, you should be familiar with it: LDL. The lower the better.

Ask your doctor for a lipid analysis, a fancy name for a blood test that checks those cholesterol guises. Your doctor will focus on the LDL results. If your LDL is less than 100, you are at low risk for heart disease. In most cases, you will need medication to lower your LDL.

Triglycerides

YOUR LIPID ANALYSIS will also test for another fat-like substance traveling in your blood called "triglycerides." In most cases, having high triglycerides means you are overweight and inactive. Other things can raise triglycerides, like smoking and consuming alcohol, and taking in too many carbohydrates. High triglycerides, like high LDL, put you at a higher risk for heart disease. You have the power to lower your triglycerides, because the way you live affects the level. Most people can lower triglycerides by losing weight and becoming more active. You want your triglycerides to be below 150.

THE HEALTHY WEIGH: Know your LDL cholesterol, triglycerides, blood pressure, and Body Mass Index.

Blood Pressure

BLOOD PRESSURE IS ACTUALLY the pressure of your blood as it courses through your arteries. Lucky for you, the test is cheap, easy, and painless. Fast, too, and it should be done every time you visit your doctor. Best blood pressure is 120 (or less) /80 (or less).

Obesity

HOW CAN YOU FIGURE OUT if you are carrying around extra pounds? Look at the ratio of your weight to your height. This is called "Body Mass Index" (BMI), and if you take a look at this table, you can make the calculation.

	Normal						Overweight					Obese						
BMI	19	20	21	22	23	24	25	26	27	28	29	30	31	32	33	34	35	36
Height (inches)												**Body Weight** (pounds)						
58	91	96	100	105	110	115	119	124	129	134	138	143	148	153	158	162	167	172
59	94	99	104	109	114	119	124	128	133	138	143	148	153	158	163	168	173	178
60	97	102	107	112	118	123	128	133	138	143	148	153	158	163	168	174	179	184
61	100	106	111	116	122	127	132	137	143	148	153	158	164	169	174	180	185	190
62	104	109	115	120	126	131	136	142	147	153	158	164	169	175	180	186	191	196
63	107	113	118	124	130	135	141	146	152	158	163	169	175	180	186	191	197	203
64	110	116	122	128	134	140	145	151	157	163	169	174	180	186	192	197	204	209
65	114	120	126	132	138	144	150	156	162	168	174	180	186	192	198	204	210	216
66	118	124	130	136	142	148	155	161	167	173	179	186	192	198	204	210	216	223
67	121	127	134	140	146	153	159	166	172	178	185	191	198	204	211	217	223	230
68	125	131	138	144	151	158	164	171	177	184	190	197	203	210	216	223	230	236
69	128	135	142	149	155	162	169	176	182	189	196	203	209	216	223	230	236	243
70	132	139	146	153	160	167	174	181	188	195	202	209	216	222	229	236	243	250
71	136	143	150	157	165	172	179	186	193	200	208	215	222	229	236	243	250	257
72	140	147	154	162	169	177	184	191	199	206	213	221	228	235	242	250	258	265
73	144	151	159	166	174	182	189	197	204	212	219	227	235	242	250	257	265	272
74	148	155	163	171	179	186	194	202	210	218	225	233	241	249	256	264	272	280
75	152	160	168	176	184	192	200	208	216	224	232	240	248	256	264	272	279	287
76	156	164	172	180	189	197	205	213	221	230	238	246	254	263	271	279	287	295

And now for some exciting new markers:

Homocysteine

WE ALL REMEMBER when cholesterol was an unfamiliar word, and we all know where that went. So it shouldn't surprise you that another new word has come on the scene, and, as luck would have it, another one that would stump the national spelling bee champ. The word is *"homocysteine"* (pronounced homo-SIS-teen), and like cholesterol, it's circulating in your blood right this minute. When it goes hand-in-hand with high LDL, it is associated with heart disease.

Like cholesterol, homocysteine can be measured in the blood,

			Extreme Obesity															
37	38	39	40	41	42	43	44	45	46	47	48	49	50	51	52	53	54	BMI
																		Height
177	181	186	191	196	201	205	210	215	220	224	229	234	239	244	248	253	258	58
183	188	193	198	203	208	212	217	222	227	232	237	242	247	252	257	262	267	59
189	194	199	204	209	215	220	225	230	235	240	245	250	255	261	266	271	276	60
195	201	206	211	217	222	227	232	238	243	248	254	259	264	269	275	280	285	61
202	207	213	218	224	229	235	240	246	251	256	262	267	273	278	284	289	295	62
208	214	220	225	231	237	242	248	254	259	265	270	278	282	287	293	299	304	63
215	221	227	232	238	244	250	256	262	267	273	279	285	291	296	302	308	314	64
222	228	234	240	246	252	258	264	270	276	282	288	294	300	306	312	318	324	65
229	235	241	247	253	260	266	272	278	284	291	297	303	309	315	322	328	334	66
236	242	249	255	261	268	274	280	287	293	299	306	312	319	325	331	338	344	67
243	249	256	262	269	276	282	289	295	302	308	315	322	328	335	341	348	354	68
250	257	263	270	277	284	291	297	304	311	318	324	331	338	345	351	358	365	69
257	264	271	278	285	292	299	306	313	320	327	334	341	348	355	362	369	376	70
265	272	279	286	293	301	308	315	322	329	338	343	351	358	365	372	379	386	71
272	279	287	294	302	309	316	324	331	338	346	353	361	368	375	383	390	397	72
280	288	295	302	310	318	325	333	340	348	355	363	371	378	386	393	401	408	73
287	295	303	311	319	326	334	342	350	358	365	373	381	389	396	404	412	420	74
295	303	311	319	327	335	343	351	359	367	375	383	391	399	407	415	423	431	75
304	312	320	328	336	344	353	361	369	377	385	394	402	410	418	426	435	443	76

high levels have been found in people with heart disease, and high levels in people without heart disease are at an increased risk of developing it.

But there is a big, big difference between these two spelling bee monsters. While cholesterol is old hat at this point (the focus is now on LDL cholesterol), homocysteine is decidedly not. Cholesterol is a mature adult; homocysteine is just a baby, and there is much less hard information available about it. For instance, while it makes sense to lower homocysteine, we don't yet have studies showing that doing so reduces heart disease. What we do know is that it's a tiny particle that can do big, big damage by irritating blood vessels (not a good thing), which can lead to blockages, even strokes (definitely not good).

But already there's a lot of exciting stuff out there, and the most exciting of all is that for most people it's really easy to deal with high homocysteine levels. It's even easy to keep them from becoming high in the first place. How? With folic acid, a B vitamin found in fruits, vegetables, and starchy beans — in other words, the DASH diet. In fact, folic acid is so important that grains are being fortified with it. Besides all the good the DASH diet does for blood pressure, it also lowers homocysteine levels.

C-Reactive Protein (CRP)

C-REACTIVE PROTEIN (CRP) forms in the blood when inflammation is present in the body.

CRP in your blood means your body is working hard to fight some type of unhealthy intrusion. We call this work a low-grade inflammation, and it can be caused by bacteria, or a virus, gum disease, even cigarette smoking. You may feel healthy, because everything is happening silently, behind the scenes.

CRP in the blood can be measured with a test, which is fortunate, since elevated CRP can predict heart disease years in advance. In the ongoing Women's Health Study, an elevated level of CRP was actually a better predictor of risk for heart disease than elevated LDL. So we see that the presence of inflammation is a risk factor for heart disease, and may well be why taking aspirin reduces that risk.

By the way, when you ask for the test, make sure to specify "high sensitivity CRP.'" Sometimes it's called "hsCRP," or "Cardio CRP," names for the same test. Nothing is simple.

GORY DETAILS
OF SERVING SIZES

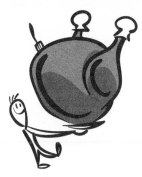

DASH WAS A FEEDING STUDY in which people were given a certain amount of food to eat. This guaranteed that the researchers could analyze results with precision and accuracy. However, when you're talking about a "free-range" population, people who are living on their own and not being fed by researchers, it's a lot harder to discuss and describe what they are eating. Which brings us to serving sizes, an attempt to "standardize" things to some extent.

To add to the confusion, serving sizes are governed by three completely different, separate, well-respected agencies in these United States of America, and the serving sizes vary depending on the agency. First is the Food Pyramid of the USDA (United States Department of Agriculture). Second is the "commonly consumed serving size" of the FDA (Food and Drug Administration) on the food label's Nutrition Facts. And third is the "exchange list" of the ADA's (American Dietetic Association and the American Diabetes Association). All their serving sizes are different, and they've driven us crazy. So we say: Unless, for particular medical reasons you have to standardize your serving sizes, just eat a piece of fruit at every meal, and don't worry about its being any particular size. Is there any chance that you are overeating fruit? Virtually none. There are guidelines for serving sizes for both raw and cooked fruits, but bottom line is — eat fruit at every meal and for a snack.

If all of this sounds a little bit casual to you and you want more specifics, here they are. We include the serving sizes used in the DASH diet. They are also the ones we used in the recipe section, Preparing the Best Foods on Earth.

THE HEALTHY WEIGH: Don't be confused about serving sizes. Ask a dietician to personalize your serving size goals.

Fruits	6 ounces fruit juice 1 medium fruit 1/2 cup fresh (cut up), frozen or canned 1/4 cup dried fruit
Vegetables	1 cup raw 1/2 cup cooked 6 ounces vegetable juice
Dairy	8 ounces low-fat or fat-free milk 1 cup low-fat or fat-free yogurt 1 1/2 ounces low-fat or fat-free cheese
Grains	1 slice bread 1/2 cup dry cereal 1/2 cup cooked cereal, rice, potatoes, pasta
Meat/Poultry/Fish	3 ounces, cooked
Nuts, Seeds, Legumes	1/3 cup nuts 2 tablespoons seeds 1/2 cup cooked legumes
Fats	1 teaspoon oil, margarine, butter, or mayonnaise 1 tablespoon "reduced fat" or "lite" margarine, mayonnaise, or whipped butter 2 teaspoons peanut butter 1 tablespoon salad dressing 2 tablespoons "reduced fat" or "lite" salad dressing

STARCHES AND WEIGHT LOSS

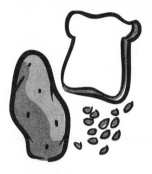

YOU MAY HAVE NOTICED that the DASH diet doesn't have a "starches" category. Well, maybe you didn't notice, and maybe you don't care, but trust us. There isn't. Now it may be that, when you think of starch, you think of dropping off your shirts at the laundry, but the starches we have in mind are plant foods. Of course they're included in the DASH diet because they're healthy, excellent foods — some of the best on earth. Here they make appearances as grains, legumes, and vegetables.

All grains (including bread, cereal, pasta, and all the things we've discussed already) are starches. So are legumes. As for vegetables, there's a whole category called "starchy," very familiar ones like peas, corn, limas, potatoes, sweet potatoes, and winter squash. Winter squashes have a hard exterior, as opposed to a soft, nonstarchy squash like zucchini. They have wonderful names like acorn, hubbard, and butternut.

The great thing about starches is that they are a major source of energy, which we need in order to work, play with the grandkids, clean the house, wash the car, work in the garden, bowl, run, bicycle, and move around.

So where's the weight loss? You promised us a weight loss discussion! Yes, we did, and here it is.

Because starches are such an excellent source of energy, if you eat too much of them, you will have so much excess energy you'll explode into teeny tiny pieces. Just kidding. But if you overeat starches, you'll gain weight. As a matter of fact, if you overeat anything, you will gain weight.

The flip side of all of this is that you may be avoiding starches because you have heard they cause weight gain. The truth is it's overeating itself that causes weight gain. The point here is that you don't want to avoid starches, because you'll be missing the health wallop of grains, starchy vegetables, and legumes. They've been around for a long time, and they've never gone out of style.

THE HEALTHY WEIGH:
You can lose weight and eat starches! Just eat the right amount. A dietitian can help you do that.

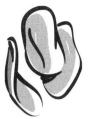

Fake Starches

SNACK FOODS LIKE POTATO CHIPS, "breakfast-in-a-bar" foods, candy bars that masquerade as health bars for women, sweetened cereals (is there one called "Choc-o-Matic"?) — all these have one thing in common. Somewhere buried deep in their ancestry is a grain. So yes, they are technically starches. But time, evolution, and technology have conspired to make them valueless from a food standpoint. Walk on by.

GRAPEFRUIT ADVICE

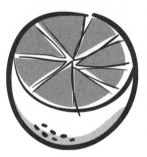

THE DASH PATTERN includes lots of fruits. Rumor has it that one fruit, grapefruit, can cause problems. The truth is that grapefruit in any form — fresh, juiced, or supplements — increases the concentration in your blood of certain medications. Something in grapefruit can alter the way the liver processes these medications. One type of medication affected by grapefruit are "statins," a class of medications that lowers cholesterol. You may experience muscle pain, lightheadedness, or toxic blood levels when you combine statins and grapefruit. If you are taking any medications at all, check with your doctor or pharmacist to make sure they dance well with grapefruit/grapefruit juice. Then you'll know whether or not you have to eliminate it from your diet. While you're at it, find out if there are any other foods you should avoid because of your medications.

IN A NUTSHELL:
Start today! Know that DASH is
THE BEST DIET ON EARTH!

9

STAYING
ON TRACK

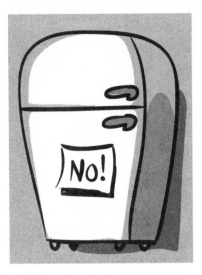

YOU'VE BEEN DOING FINE with all of this, we know you have: fruits, vegetables, low-fat dairy, whole grains — maybe a few nuts in there somewhere. But lately, something has changed. You don't know what, exactly, but old habits seem to be rearing their ugly heads. Well, let's revisit our co-author and resident dietitian, Francine Grabowski, whose professional life is dedicated to helping real people, you, make the changes you need to take care of yourself and then to stay on track. ★ **Francine Grabowski:** HOW EXACTLY DO YOU DO THIS? I can't give you the answer. What I can give you is the time and space to think about what will work for you. I can share with you the stories of people in similar situations. These stories will help you figure out what is preventing you from moving forward. We can all learn lessons from patients who believed in themselves despite the slips and the falls, who got themselves moving again and back on track. They are inspiring.

"This is real," and "I get it."

JOHN CAME IN FOR HIS SECOND VISIT. He didn't say much, but he did bring in his homework assignment. And he had lost weight. From the homework assignment, the weight loss and his answers to my questions, I could tell that he was following his meal plan. He absolutely knew what he had to do and was doing it.

I was very excited — more than he was, as a matter of fact — and told him how hard it is for people to reach this level of accomplishment. When I asked him the secret of his success, he answered, "Two three-word sentences." He explained that, during his last visit to his doctor, he was told he had no choice but to make changes. And then the doctor said, "This is real." John explained that those three words led him to make an appointment with me, and, having listened to my strategies, he understood the game plan. With no fanfare whatsoever, he added, "I get it." Again — three words.

After he left, I thought about the power of his conviction, the strength of simplicity and the power of getting to the heart of the issue. To this day, when I think of him and his three-word sentences, I am filled with strength. Try it for yourself: when you find yourself drifting, think of the words "this is real." They will bring you back.

Three Little Words

THREE LITTLE WORDS. THAT'S ALL IT TAKES. Just three little words. If this were a song, the words would be "I love you," but this isn't a song. It's about strength, simplicity, and things to keep you on track.

Let's look at other "three little words."

The "Aha!" Moment

LISA KNEW SHE WAS IN IT FOR THE LONG HAUL. She told me how much she loved her home and how she loved to keep it clean, but instead of doing those things she loved, she was visiting me and planning meals — something she did not enjoy as much as beautifying her home. So why was she doing this? Seven years ago, at the age of 34, she developed diabetes during her pregnancy — "gestational diabetes." It went away after the birth of her child, but she was told it would most likely come back, particularly if she gained weight.

She did, and it did. When she came to see me, she had just been diagnosed with diabetes, as well as high blood pressure, and high cholesterol. (This trio is often found together.) She knew she had to lose weight, eat right, and exercise. She knew "this is real."

She told me that, in spite of an unwavering commitment, this was hard to do every day. Then she said, "You know what has helped me? My 'best friend,' Oprah Winfrey. She had a program on the 'aha!' moment."

An "aha!" moment is that instant when you truly realize what you are doing. Call it a "reality check." Lisa might have an "aha!" moment when she buys food, or when she orders at a restaurant. It hits her that this is not something she wants to be eating.

In order to have an "aha!" moment, you have to be awake, alert, aware. You simply cannot afford the luxury of cruising along on automatic pilot and suddenly realize you've eaten an entire serving of something you never meant to order in the first place. When she puts anything in her mouth, she thinks first. She described to me how she picks up a new frozen food, looks at the label and it hits her; "There's a lot of fat in here."

It is possible to become more awake, alert, and aware. Spend more time with like-minded people, maybe join a support group like Weight Watchers or Overeaters Anonymous. Working with a dietitian or taking classes will also increase your awake/alert/aware level.

The rewards of "aha!" moments, of being awake/alert/aware, do much more for you than improve your health. They help you savor and appreciate the here-and-now, which is a great way to live.

"I am courageous."

LEARN HOW TO SAY THESE WORDS TO YOURSELF, because they are true and you should know that. Another "three little words."

It's not uncommon to feel disillusioned that you aren't making progress every day, but keep in mind that the work you are doing to take care of yourself takes courage. Making changes takes courage! You probably never thought of yourself as courageous, but trust me. You are. Working every single day to be a healthier person in a world that is conspiring against you all the time — well, that sounds like a pretty good definition of courageous to me.

Imagine if every restaurant served small portions on small plates, if every dinner party you went to featured only the kinds of foods you are trying to focus on, if everyone in your neighborhood went out together to walk before going to work. Imagine if your workplace gave you time off during the day to exercise. Usually that privilege is saved for the prison population.

But the world isn't like that, is it? So you can see the courage it takes to make these tough decisions in the real world (not to mention a world with unexpected health detours). And to stay pleasant and positive while you're making those decisions. Your capacity for enjoyment is intact even as you keep your "eye on the prize." You are focused but not over-focused. You enjoy your family, your friendships, your hobbies. You appreciate the little things — as the song says, "raindrops on roses and whiskers on kittens. . . ."

Now that's courageous.

Be Kind to Yourself

PAT WAS BEGINNING HER SESSION with all the things she had done wrong since I had last seen her. She over-ate, she did not exercise, she didn't follow her meal plan, and she didn't eat vegetables or fruit. She was more than disappointed with herself. She was unforgiving, quick to judge, harsh, cold, and critical. No doubt about it, she believed she was a failure. I asked her what she would do if her young daughter had recited a list of failures. She thought about that and said that she would help her daughter see things differently. She would offer caring words of trust and concern. She would make sure her daughter knew that success was around the corner. In other words, Pat would be kind.

I suggested to Pat that she be similarly kind to herself. I pointed out that this would help her return to creative problem solving and let her move forward.

Plan, Plan, Plan

HOW ARE YOU GOING TO MAKE GOOD FOOD CHOICES? Where are you going to get your fruit, your vegetables? Have a game plan. A plan for when you eat at fancy restaurants, a plan for when you eat at fast food places, a plan for when you are running late at work. A plan for when you work late on Tuesdays. And if you are caught without a plan — say you are sitting on a runway for three hours and all you can find to eat is a mayonnaise packet in the seat back in front of you — well, let this remind you to have a plan the next time. You can accumulate dozens of plans for all the wonderful unexpected and challenging situations that occur in your life. Don't leave home without one!

Practice, Practice, Practice

JUDITH IS AN EXTRAORDINARY FIRST GRADE TEACHER. Her face beams with the excitement of joyful teaching. She is upbeat and playful, but she gets very serious when she discusses her 27-pound weight loss. "If you want to do something right," she says, "you have to practice, practice, practice. Whether it is playing the piano or learning to read or planning meals, it's all the same. But like I tell my kids, you get very good at what you practice."

Be Kind To Others

IF YOU FIND THAT YOU ARE BEMOANING your "fate," expand your reach. Do something for somebody else. If you help someone else, that is time well spent, as well as time you won't be thinking about yourself, about what you can and cannot eat. When you do something for someone else, you actually feel better about yourself. Life is funny that way.

Let It Grow

HAVE YOU EVER MET PEOPLE who are changing the way they eat? All they talk about is food. They eat, breathe, and sleep "The Zone" or "Atkins" or "vegetarian." The truth is, in the beginning, you need to spend a lot of time practicing and mastering. And sometimes that time includes "converting" — you want to share the good news with those around you. But there is more to life than food. Don't just sit there and dwell on what you can and cannot eat. Now that you have practiced, practiced, practiced, and this new skill is second nature, move on. Let yourself grow. Live life to the fullest. Be loving, be attentive to your family and friends, be active in your community. Be physically active. Join a team, coach a team, start a club, advocate for better mass transportation. Learn to play bridge, read poetry, write poetry.

If you have made the necessary changes, you've discovered you are NOT an old dog who cannot learn new tricks. You can do it! You can master whatever you set your sights on. Let it grow.

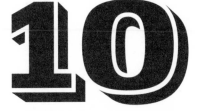

10

FREQUENTLY ASKED QUESTIONS ("FAQ'S")

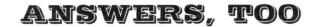

ANSWERS, TOO

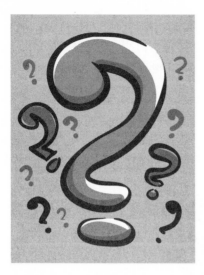

IF THESE QUESTIONS SPEAK TO YOU, you have a lot of company. They are questions that we've been asked (professionally and nonprofessionally) over and over again. ⭐ **Q: Can't I just take a vitamin instead of eating fruits and vegetables? A:** There is no "magic pill," vitamin or otherwise. Whatever pills are invented, there will never be a true substitute for the wonderful health mystery we call food. ⭐ **Q: How come my baby carrots sometimes taste like the middle of the tree? A:** Because they are not "baby carrots," sweet and tender. They are actually old carrots that have been cut to look small. Ha ha, the joke's on you. Read the package carefully so you know what you're getting. ⭐ **Q: How do I know a package of pre-washed lettuce is fresh? A:** Hold it up to the light and you'll see the date. Tip (close your eyes, supermarket produce people): The freshest bags are at the back of the shelf. And fresh lettuce looks green and vibrant, not brown or yellowed. ⭐ **Q: What are "greens"? A:** A nickname for dark, leafy green vegetables such as spinach, kale, collard, chard, escarole, beet greens, turnip greens, mustard greens.

Q: What do I do with fresh greens?

A: Leafy greens should be carefully washed several times in clean water. Lift the leaves each time to make sure all the sand/dirt is out. Discard the bruised leaves, dry the greens, and store them in a plastic bag with some paper towels to soak up the excess moisture, and put into the refrigerator, where they'll keep for several days.

Q: How much fresh greens should I buy?

A: One pound of fresh, uncooked greens makes two-to-three cooked servings.

Q: How can I pick the freshest greens?

A: Look for leaves that are crisp (not wilted), deep green, with no trace of yellow. The smaller the leaves, the milder the taste.

Q: I don't want to wash all those greens. Any ideas?

A: Try frozen.

Q: How do you cut up winter squash? It's so hard!

A: It's hard, all right, in both senses of the word. You need a good, sharp knife, a steady hand, and a valiant heart. If you are knife-shy, buy frozen. Or you might try cooking it whole, in the oven, and remove the seeds later. A cooked squash is easy to cut. And your produce section may be a "cut above the rest" (ha ha) and have fresh, peeled, cut-up acorn (and other) squash just waiting for you to take it home and cook.

Q: Can you help me get over my fear of preparing fresh vegetables?

A: Yes, indeed-y, and funny you should ask. Get yourself a bag of pre-washed baby spinach leaves. Sauté them with some chopped onion in a little spray vegetable oil, or add a small amount of water and steam them. They'll cook in a jiffy and taste like a dream.

Q: Does ketchup count as a vegetable?

A: What are you, a hold-over from the Reagan administration? Ketchup? A vegetable? Are you kidding? (Lots of question marks considering this is an "answer," but you get the idea.) No, ketchup does not count as a vegetable. One of us calls it a sweetener; the other calls it a topping. Take your choice.

Q: I eat lots of vegetables. At lunch every day I have a pickle with my hamburger, and I have lettuce and tomato on the burger. Pretty good, don't you think?

A: No, as a matter of fact, we don't. These are mere "token vegetables." Sounds like you believe that ketchup is a vegetable.

Q: Should I eat organic produce?

A: If your store carries it, try it. Less pesticide residue. M-m-m-m, better.

Q: Do I HAVE to eat organic produce?

A: Not necessarily. You'll get that health wallop no matter what.

Q: What about the salt in canned vegetables?

A: Since "no salt added" canned vegetables are easy to find, why not go with them?

Q: What if I don't like fruits or vegetables?

A: You are at a distinct disadvantage, which you obviously realize. Think of yourself as a child learning to eat something new, and try a little bit at a time. Studies show that repeated exposure does the trick, so persevere. Good luck! We'll be thinking of you.

Q: Can I get my fruit as juice?

A: Yes, if it's 100% juice. Naturally we hope you bite into a piece of fruit from time to time.

Q: What about the sugar in canned fruit?

A: First and foremost, you want to eat fruit, and if that's the only way you'll eat it, go for it. The best thing you can do is eat a variety of fruits, including fresh, frozen, dried, and canned.

Q: Does fruit jam count as a fruit?

A: Wouldn't that be nice? But the answer, unfortunately, is "no."

Q: If I eat all those fruits, vegetables, and whole grains, won't I have gas or diarrhea?

A: A sudden shift in any eating pattern can cause this kind of disruption, as you know if you've traveled to foreign lands. In a few days, your system adapts to the new regimen. Meanwhile, be kind to yourself and take it slowly. Small steps have powerful results.

Q: Are you telling me I have to eat vegetarian?

A: No, no, no, no, no! Absolutely not! Still, if only for the sake of variety, it's kind of nice to eat vegetarian every once in a while. Pasta's always good.

Q: What can I do about the fact that vegetable/grain meals taste bland?

A: Sounds like your tastebuds could use some pizzazz. Experiment with some new recipes and flavors. Check the recipe section at the back of this book, "Preparing the Best Foods on Earth."

Q: **What are whole grain foods?**
A: Nothing fancy — just food that comes to you without any tricks: corn, oats, barley, rice (both brown and wild), and rye. AND foods made with whole wheat flour.

Q: **How do I know a bread is a whole grain bread?**
A: Is there a label? What does it say? Remember, you're in good shape if the bread label lists whole wheat or rye as the first ingredient. Sometimes there's a shortcut, which is the word "whole" written in big letters on the package. If you have lots of time on your hands, maybe vacationing in the supermarket, you might look at the health claim on the package: "Diets rich in whole grain foods and other plant foods low in saturated fat and cholesterol, may help reduce the risk of heart disease and certain cancers." Wordy? Indeed. But it guarantees that you're holding a whole grain product in your hands.

Q: **What are some whole grain cereals?**
A: Think retro. Golden Oldies are in when it comes to whole grain cereals. Some products that can claim "whole grain fame": Cheerios, Wheaties, Whole Grain Total, Shredded Wheat, and Raisin Bran.

Q: **How do I know which whole grain breads taste best?**
A: Nothing beats a taste test. Ask around — maybe someone has some recommendations. After all, you'd ask around if you needed a dentist, wouldn't you?

Q: **What about "lite" breads?**
A: Lucky you! Lite breads come in whole grain (such as Manischewitz Seeded Lite Rye), which have a very nice taste. So if you're looking for a way to have your bread and eat it too, try lite whole grain. These breads are reduced in calories. In some cases, two slices have the same calories as a single slice of regular bread.

Q: **But I don't eat bread! How am I going to get my whole grains?**
A: How about whole grain pastas? They offer a good chance to have whole grains. Try the smaller pastas for taste and texture. Keep testing different brands and shapes until you find a pasta you can be proud of.

Q: **Do I have to go to a health food store to buy whole wheat pasta?**
A: We hope not. We hope your grocery store carries whole grains and lots of fruits and vegetables. By the way, there is a grocery store in certain states that is truly innovative in whole food selections: "Trader Joe's." Look for one around you. You will be in for a treat.

Q: You win. I'm convinced to go for whole grains. Can I substitute brown rice for white rice in my casseroles?

A: By all means; that's a really healthy change! While you're at it, try wild rice, too.

Q: What do you do with wild rice?

A: Go wild, of course! Its nutty texture and wonderful flavor enhances all your rice dishes. Experiment!

Q: I shy away from whole grain rice because it takes too long to cook. Suggestions?

A: A great tasting brown rice that takes about the same amount of cooking time as white is Uncle Ben's Brown Rice Natural Whole Grain (Ready in 30 Minutes). More convenient but, frankly, not quite as tasty, is Uncle Ben's Instant Brown Rice. Barley, by the way, also comes in a quick-cooking variety that is every bit as good as the longer-cooking: Mother's 100% Natural Wholegrain Barley.

Q: Doesn't it seem like all these fruits, vegetables, and whole grains are an awful lot to eat?

A: It looks like you're eating more food and it feels like you're eating more food, but, as far as your body is concerned, you're not.

Q: How about the Food Guide Pyramid we've gotten used to? What does all of this have to do with that?

A: It's exactly what the pyramid calls for, with small modifications — namely, that you eat even more fruits and vegetables than suggested, and you make better food choices overall. That is, whole grains from the grain section, plant fats from the fats section, and lean and extra lean from the meat section. That's what the original research says. On the other hand, the pyramid might benefit from a little redistricting. Besides having more emphasis on fruits and vegetables, it could use a separate area for nuts and seeds, and for starchy beans.

Q: I like regular milk. There is no way I could drink non-fat milk. Any ideas?

A: You are in for a treat. Milk manufacturers have found a way to make nonfat milk taste like 2% milk. (By the way, 2% is very close to the rich full taste of whole milk.) How do they do it? By adding fibers called gums, maybe a little more protein or maybe a little more calcium. There is no one name for this milk. Check out your milk department and look for something that is advertised something like this: "nonfat with the rich taste of 2%."

Q: What's so important about calcium?

A: We need calcium for healthy bones, strong bones. We build these strong bones only until our early 30's. After that, we are trying to protect what we have, and calcium is essential. Milk is the best source of calcium.

Q: What if I don't like milk at all?

A: If you're the same person who doesn't like fruits or vegetables, you're really in a mess, aren't you? Start with four ounces of low-fat or fat-free milk at each meal. Eat a little yogurt, have a little low-fat or fat-free cheese. You'll get there.

Q: What can I do? My cafeteria does not carry low-fat (let alone fat-free) milk.

A: Get up a petition! If enough people want it, they'll carry it.

Q: What is a good low-fat/ fat-free cheese?

A: We like Alpine Lace, Cabot, Kraft, and Jarlsberg Lite Reduced Fat.

Q: It's holiday time! I look forward to this all year! Are you suggesting that I give up my traditional holiday treats?

A: Of course not. Eat and enjoy. We are, however, suggesting that you not overeat. When you really, truly binge, you feel really, truly terrible anyway. Just go easy.

Q: How can I lose weight?

A: Check out **THE HEALTHY WEIGH** throughout this book.

Q: I've heard that starches cause weight gain. Is that true?

A: Starches don't cause weight gain. Overeating and under-moving cause weight gain.

Q: What about these fat-free cakes and cookies I keep hearing about?

A: They are popular, all right, but all they do is keep you from eating a healthy snack. They can really put weight on you, too, if you eat a lot of them.

Q: Can I eat sweets?

A: Of course you can — but should you? If you are eating plenty of fruits, vegetables, low-fat dairy, and whole grains, then by all means, yes. If you have time. And, of course, they can put weight on you, too.

Q: What about fat?

A: Avoid the biggies — saturated and trans fats. Remember, as far as your body is concerned, trans fats (think "hydrogenated and partially hydrogenated" vegetable oils) act like saturated fat. Pretty unappealing, don't you think?

Q: Are there margarines with no trans fat?
A: There are, indeed: Smart Beat, Olivio, Brummel & Brown, Promise Buttery Lite, Fleischmann's Premium Blend Squeeze. Taste test to find the one you like best.

Q: What about the margarines that lower LDL cholesterol?
A: You mean Benecol and Take Control. If you use margarine and have high LDL cholesterol, you might want to give them a try.

Q: Can I use salt?
A: Sure, in small amounts. It only takes a small amount of salt to give the flavor you want. What is a small amount? Put a quarter of a teaspoon of salt in a shaker and use for the whole day.

Q: How do I know a packaged food is low in sodium?
A: Look at the Nutrition Facts. Make sure you have something that is less than 5% Daily Value for Sodium.

Q: If I'm going to follow the DASH diet, do I have to give up caffeine?
A: Participants were allowed three caffeinated beverages per day (coffee or tea). If they could do it, so can you.

Q: How about alcohol? If I'm going to follow the DASH diet, does that mean no drinks?
A: DASH participants were allowed two alcoholic drinks each day (beer, white wine, liquor). And we say again: If they could do it, so can you.

Q: I'm a slug. What can I do to take more steps?
A: Get a pedometer. Just wearing it will make you take more steps. If weight loss is something you're looking at, you have no choice but to get moving.

Q: What can I do? I have tried and tried, but I just can't do it!
A: You get "E" for "Effort," anyway. It may be that you're just not ready. Pick something you can do, maybe fruit with every meal. This time next year, who knows? You could be giving lectures on this.

Q: How about these high-protein diets?
A: There is no connection between high-protein diets and health. These diets are not exactly based on the Best Foods on Earth, are they? So you won't be getting their protection from heart disease, blood pressure, cancer, and diabetes.

Q: Will all of this be worth it to me?

A: You already know about the remarkable long-term benefits of THE BEST DIET ON EARTH. Chances are you will feel better, too, and your body will thank you again and again.

FOOD RECORD:
What did I eat? When did I eat it?

MORNING:

TIME OF DAY	FOOD	HOW MUCH?

AFTERNOON:

TIME OF DAY	FOOD	HOW MUCH?

EVENING:

TIME OF DAY	FOOD	HOW MUCH?

FOOD RECORD:
What did I eat? When did I eat it?

MORNING:

TIME OF DAY	FOOD	HOW MUCH?

AFTERNOON:

TIME OF DAY	FOOD	HOW MUCH?

EVENING:

TIME OF DAY	FOOD	HOW MUCH?

FOOD RECORD:
What did I eat? When did I eat it?

MORNING:

TIME OF DAY	FOOD	HOW MUCH?

AFTERNOON:

TIME OF DAY	FOOD	HOW MUCH?

EVENING:

TIME OF DAY	FOOD	HOW MUCH?

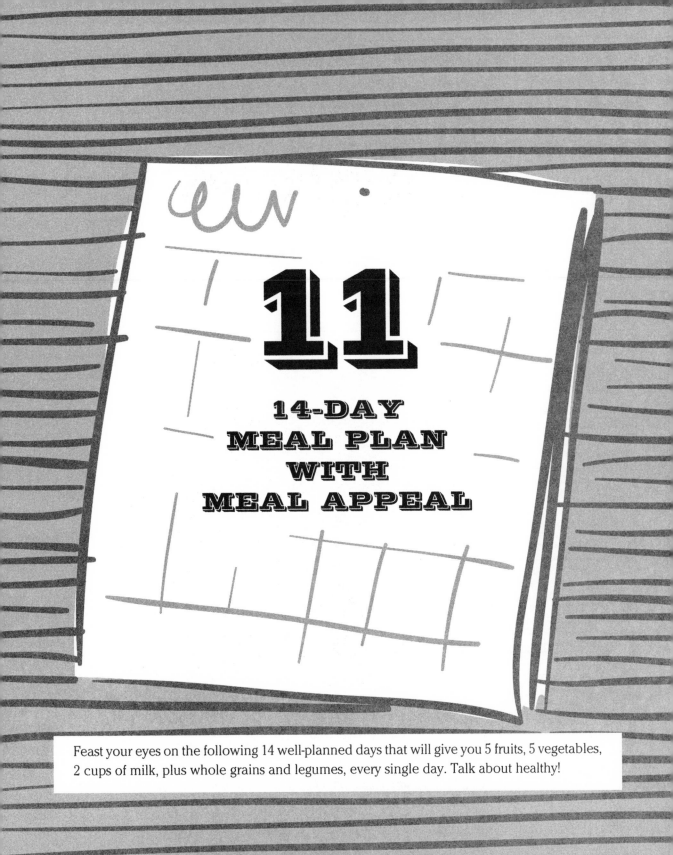

11

14-DAY MEAL PLAN WITH MEAL APPEAL

Feast your eyes on the following 14 well-planned days that will give you 5 fruits, 5 vegetables, 2 cups of milk, plus whole grains and legumes, every single day. Talk about healthy!

Day 1

Food	Amount	Grain	Veg	Fruit	Dairy	Meat	Nuts	Fats	Sweets
BREAKFAST									
Orange juice	6 ounces			1					
Eggo Whole Grain pancakes	2	1							
Fat-free milk	8 ounces				1				
REAL FRUIT TOPPING	1/2 cup			1					
Lite margarine	1 TBSP.							1	
LUNCH									
12 BEAN SOUP	2 cups		2				2	1/2	
Whole grain dinner roll	1	1							
Apricot nectar	6 ounces			1					
DINNER									
TERRIFIC TILAPIA	3 ounces		1			3			
Whole grain pasta	1 cup	2							
BROCCOLI CAULIFLOWER RIOT	1 cup		2						
UNBEATABLE BEET GREENS	1 cup		2						
GRANNY GRAPES AND YOGURT	1 cup			1	1				
Lite margarine	1 TBSP.							1	
SNACK									
Crispy apple	1			1					
Fat-free milk	4 ounces								

Note that the recipes in capital letters may be found in the following chapter,
PREPARING THE BEST FOODS ON EARTH: DAY-BY-DAY RECIPES

Day 2

Food	Amount	Grain	Veg	Fruit	Dairy	Meat	Nuts	Fats	Sweets
BREAKFAST									
Orange juice	6 ounces			1					
DAILY EGGS	1/4 recipe		1			1			
Whole grain bread	1 slice	1							
Fat-free milk	8 ounces				1				
Lite margarine							1		
LUNCH									
ADVENTUROUS SALAD	3 cups		3						
With melon	1 cup			1					
OUR FAVORITE OIL AND VINEGAR DRESSING	1 TBSP.							1	
Hummus	1/4 cup						1	1	
Baked corn chips	1 ounce	1							
Pineapple juice	6 ounces			1					
DINNER									
"MEATLOAF" (VEG & TURKEY LOAF)	3 ounces		1			3		1	
MASHED POTATOES & CAULIFLOWER	1 cup		2						
RED & GREEN	1 cup		2						
APPLE PIELESS	1/4 recipe			1					
Fat-free milk	8 ounces				1				
SNACK									
Banana	1			1					
whole grain crackers	about 10	2							

Day 3

Food	Amount	Grain	Veg	Fruit	Dairy	Meat	Nuts	Fats	Sweets
BREAKFAST									
Grapefruit juice	6 ounces			1					
DAILY EGGS	1/4 recipe		1			1			
Manischewitz Lite Rye	2 slices	1							
Fat-free milk	8 ounces				1				
Banana	1 small			1					
Lite margarine	1 TBSP.							1	
LUNCH									
"MEATLOAF" sandwich*									
"MEATLOAF" (VEG. & TURKEY)	2 ounces		1			2		1	
Whole grain bread	2 slices	2							
Mustard									
Baby carrots	1 cup		1						
Applesauce	1/2 cup			1					
Fat-free milk	8 ounces				1				
DINNER									
LIMA DREAMS	1 cup						2		
GREENS AND WHEAT	1 cup	2	1						
ZESTY ORANGE DESSERT	1/2 recipe			1					
Salad	1 cup		1						
OUR FAVORITE OIL AND VINEGAR DRESSING	1 TBSP.							1	
SNACK									
Warm peaches	1/2 cup			1					

*Leftover

Day 4

Food	Amount	Grain	Veg	Fruit	Dairy	Meat	Nuts	Fats	Sweets
BREAKFAST									
Grapefruit	1/2			1					
DAILY EGGS	1/4 recipe		1			1			
Lite whole wheat english muffin	1	1							
Fat-free milk	8 ounces				1				
Lite margarine	1 TBSP.							1	
LUNCH									
Salad	2 cups		2						
Roast beef sandwich									
Roasted top loin beef	2 ounces					2			
Whole grain bread	2 slices	2							
Romaine lettuce									
Mustard									
Fat-free milk	8 ounces				1				
Canned pears	1/2 cup			1					
Dressing	1 TBSP.							1	
DINNER									
MEAL IN A BOWL	2 cups	1 1/2	1/2			3			
STRAWBERRY & SPINACH SALAD	1/4 recipe		1	1/2				1	
Mango, cut up	1/2 cup			1					
Whole-wheat roll	1	1							
SNACK									
Baked corn chips	1 ounce	1							
Ajvar	1/4 cup		1						
Apple Juice	6 ounces			1					

Day 5

Food	Amount	Grain	Veg	Fruit	Dairy	Meat	Nuts	Fats	Sweets
BREAKFAST									
Orange juice	6 ounces			1					
DAILY EGGS	1/4 recipe		1			1			
Whole grain bread	2 slices	2							
Fat-free milk	8 ounces				1				
Lite margarine	1 TBSP.							1	
LUNCH									
ADVENTUROUS SALAD	2 cups		2						
Cold chicken or turkey	2 ounces					2		2	
Mandarin oranges	1/2 cup			1					
Raisins	2 TBSP.			1/2					
Whole grain bread	1 slice	1							
Fat-free milk	8 ounces				1				
DINNER									
SHRIMP WITH TOMATOES	1 cup		1			2			
EGGPLANT RICE	1 cup	2	1						
Tender green beans	1 cup		2						
Melon slices	1 cup			1					
SNACK									
Craisins	1/4 cup			1					
Walnuts	5						1/2		

Day 6

Food	Amount	Grain	Veg	Fruit	Dairy	Meat	Nuts	Fats	Sweets
BREAKFAST									
Orange juice	6 ounces			1					
DAILY EGGS	1/4 recipe					1			
Whole grain bread	1 slice	1							
Fat-free milk	8 ounces				1				
Lite margarine	1 TBSP.							1	
LUNCH									
PERSONAL PIZZA	2	2	1/2		1				
ADVENTUROUS SALAD	2 cups		2						
With 5 almonds							1/2		
OUR FAVORITE OIL AND VINEGAR DRESSING	1 TBSP.							1	
Canned Pears	1/2 cup			1					
DINNER									
"FRIED" CHICKEN	3 ounces					3			
MANGO SLAW	2 cups		2	1					1
Corn on the cob	small	1							
Whole grain roll	small	1							
Lite margarine	1 TBSP.							1	
ROASTED PINEAPPLE SLICES	2 slices			2					

Day 7

Food	Amount	Grain	Veg	Fruit	Dairy	Meat	Nuts	Fats	Sweets
BREAKFAST									
Orange juice	6 ounces			1					
Lite whole wheat English muffin	1	1							
GORGEOUS FRUIT CUSTARD	1 cup			1/4	1/2	1/2			2
Lite margarine	1 TBSP.							1	
LUNCH									
Your favorite low-fat frozen entree		1	1			2			
Frozen vegetables (added to entree)	1 cup		2						
Fat-free milk	8 ounces				1				
Mandarin oranges	2			1					
DINNER									
VEGETARIAN-FOR-BEGINNERS PIE	1/4 pie	2			1/2		1	1	
BROCCOLI TO LIVE FOR	1 cup		2						
ADVENTUROUS SALAD	2 cups		2						
STRAWBERRY TARTAR	1/2 cup			1					
OUR FAVORITE OIL AND VINEGAR DRESSING	1 TBSP.							2	
Peach nectar	6 ounces			1					

Day 8

Food	Amount	Grain	Veg	Fruit	Dairy	Meat	Nuts	Fats	Sweets
BREAKFAST									
Orange juice	6 ounces			1					
Eggo Whole Grain Pancakes	2	1 1/2							
Fat-free milk	8 ounces				1				
REAL FRUIT TOPPING	1/2 cup			1					
LUNCH									
VEGETARIAN-FOR-BEGINNERS PIE*	1/4 pie	2			1/2		1	1	
ADVENTUROUS SALAD	2 cups		2						
With cut-up apple	1			1					
OUR FAVORITE OIL AND VINEGAR DRESSING	1 TBSP.							1	
DINNER									
CAREFREE FLOUNDER	3 ounces					3			
Baked sweet potato	small		1						
VEGETABLE GARDEN	1 cup		2						
HEARTHSIDE FRUIT	1/2 cup			1					
Whole grain bread	1 slice	1							
Lite margarine	1 TBSP.							1	
SNACK									
Fat-free milk	1/2 cup				1/2				
Dried fruit	1/4 cup			1					

*Leftover

Day 9

Food	Amount	Grain	Veg	Fruit	Dairy	Meat	Nuts	Fats	Sweets
BREAKFAST									
Orange juice	6 ounces			1					
Veggie McMuffin									
Lite whole wheat English muffin	1	1							
Low-fat cheese	1 1/2 ounces				1				
BREAKFAST VEGGIES	1/2 cup		1					1/2	
LUNCH									
12 BEAN SOUP	2 cups		2				2	1/2	
Whole grain bread	1 slice	1							
Banana	small			1					
DINNER									
HEARTY MOROCCAN CHICKEN	1/6 recipe	1	1			3	1	1	
SASSY ESCAROLE	1 cup		2					1	
ROASTED RED BEET SALAD	1 cup		2						
Frozen mixed berries	1 cup			2					
Low-fat yogurt	1 cup				1				
SNACK									
Canned fruit	1/2 cup			1					

Day 10

Food	Amount	Grain	Veg	Fruit	Dairy	Meat	Nuts	Fats	Sweets
					Servings Provided				
BREAKFAST									
Grapefruit	1/2			1					
Kashi GoLean cereal	1/2 cup	1							
Raisins	1/4 cup			1					
Fat-free milk	8 ounces				1				
Whole wheat bread	1	1							
Lite margarine	1 TBSP.							1	
LUNCH									
GAZPACHO	1 cup		1						
Roast beef sandwich									
Roast beef eye of round	2 ounces					2			
Lettuce & tomato			1/2						
Lite mayonnaise	1 TBSP.							1	
Horseradish									
Crispy apple	1			1					
Fat-free milk	8 ounces				1				
DINNER									
SAVORY SALMON	3 ounces					3			
MASHED MADNESS:									
POTATOES, SWEET POTATOES, AND CARROTS	1 cup		2						
Broccoli	1 cup		2						
Canned pears	1/2 cup			1					
SNACK									
Cranberry juice with lime slices	6 ounces			1					

Day 11

Food	Amount	Grain	Veg	Fruit	Dairy	Meat	Nuts	Fats	Sweets
BREAKFAST									
FAST AND FRUITY BREAKFAST	1 cup			1	1/2				
Whole grain bread	2 slices	2							
Lite margarine	1 TBSP.							1	
LUNCH									
Apple juice	6 ounces			1					
THE BEST SALMON SALAD	1/2 cup		1			2		1	
Whole grain crackers	about 10	2							
Canned fruit cocktail	1/2 cup			1					
DINNER									
SWEET AND SOUR PORK LOINS	3 ounces			1		3		1	
Brown rice	1 cup	2							
GREENS AND CHERRIES	1 cup		2	1					
TANGY TURNIPS	1/2 cup		1					1	
Fat-free milk	8 ounces				1				
SNACK									
Lite pudding	4 ounces				1/2				
Carrots and celery, sliced	1 cup		1						

Day 12

Food	Amount	Grain	Veg	Fruit	Dairy	Meat	Nuts	Fats	Sweets
BREAKFAST									
Orange juice	6 ounces			1					
Veggie McMuffin									
Lite whole wheat English muffin	1	1							
Cabot low-fat cheese	1 1/2 ounces				1				
BREAKFAST VEGGIES	1/2 cup		1					1	
Fat-free milk	8 ounces				1				
LUNCH									
Turkey sandwich									
Whole wheat bread	2 slices	2							
Broccoli sprouts			1/2						
SUN-DRIED TOMATO PASTE			1/2					1	
Grapes	handful			1					
Almonds	5						1/2		
Apple juice	6 ounces			1					
DINNER									
YIN YANG SOUP	about 1 cup			2					
THREE-IN-ONE: RICE, BEANS & SPINACH	1 cup	1	1				1		
QUICKIE EGGPLANT PLUS	1 cup		2						
Whole grain bread	1 slice	1							
Lite margarine	1 TBSP.							1	
SNACK									
APPLES BAKED IN BOILED CIDER	1			1					

Day 13

Food	Amount	Grain	Veg	Fruit	Dairy	Meat	Nuts	Fats	Sweets
BREAKFAST									
Orange juice	6 ounces			1					
Raisin Toast	2 slices	2							
Fat-free milk	8 ounces				1				
APPLES BAKED IN BOILED CIDER*	1			1					
Lite margarine	1 TBSP.							1	
LUNCH									
Low-sodium V8 juice	6 ounces		1						
Veggie Burger	1						2		
Whole wheat roll	1	2							
Ajvar	1/4 cup		1						
Pear	1			1					
DINNER									
UNLIKELY CHICKEN	3 ounces					3			
VEGETABLES OF SPRING	1 cup		2						
ROMANTIC GLAZED STRAWBERRIES	1/4 recipe			1					
Fat-free milk	8 ounces				1				
Salad	1 cup		1						
OUR FAVORITE OIL AND VINEGAR DRESSING	1 TBSP.							1	
SNACK									
Orange	1			1					

*Leftover

Day 14

Food	Amount	Grain	Veg	Fruit	Dairy	Meat	Nuts	Fats	Sweets
BREAKFAST									
Kashi GoLean cereal	1/2 cup	1							
Raisins	2 TBSP.			1/2					
Fat-free milk	8 ounces				1				
Banana	1			1					
LUNCH									
UNLIKELY CHICKEN*	2 ounces	2				2			
ADVENTUROUS SALAD	2 cups		2						
With cut-up apple	1			1					
Craisins	2 TBSP.			1/2					
OUR FAVORITE OIL AND VINEGAR DRESSING	1 TBSP.							1	
DINNER									
SALMON CROQUETTES	1/4 recipe		1/2			3		1	
SUCCOTASH BASH	1/2 cup		1/2				1/2		
Broccoli	1 cup		2						
Whole grain roll	1	1							
Canned lite peaches	1/2 cup			1					
Lite margarine	1 TBSP.							1	
SNACK									
Whole grain pretzels	1 ounce	1							
Lite yogurt	1				1				
Apple juice	6 ounces			1					

*Leftover

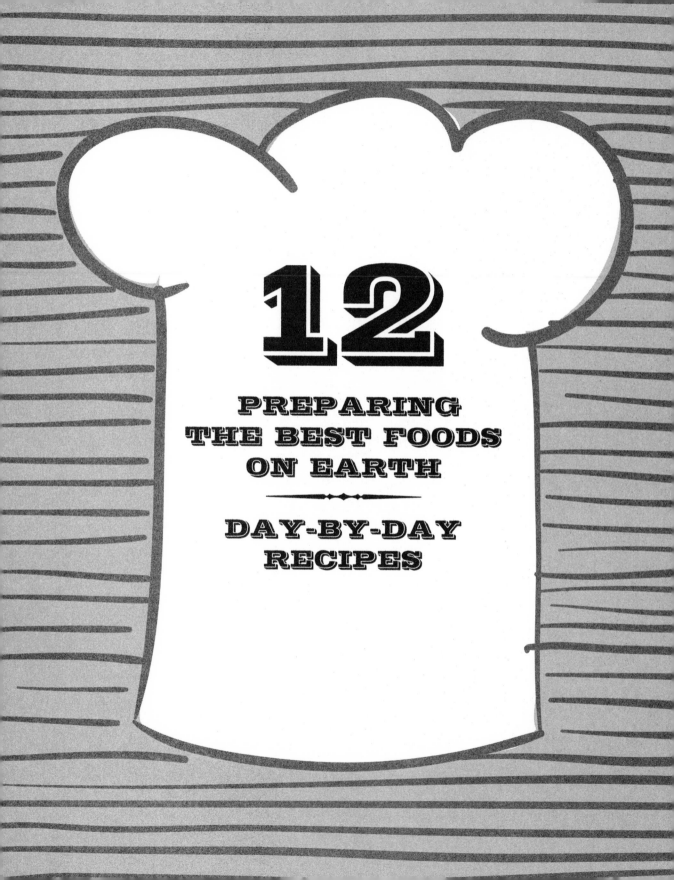

12

PREPARING THE BEST FOODS ON EARTH

DAY-BY-DAY RECIPES

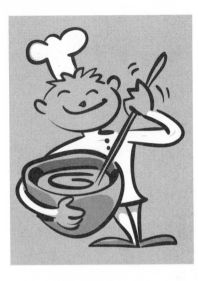

ON YOUR WAY TO HEALTHIER DAYS

EVERYTHING IN THIS BOOK is based on a wonderful study, DASH, about the benefits of foods that grow in the ground. Plants. Very, very healthy and with very, very impressive health benefits. All that's left is to prepare them for eating. ★ Now that you are about to embark on a new cooking/eating adventure, you'll be delighted at how easy it is to make room each day for the fruits, vegetables, and whole grains that are the heart of healthy DASH days. All of the following recipes are indeed healthy, tasty, and easy on your clock. ★ You'll notice that there are no lists analyzing the amounts of protein, carbohydrate, fat, sodium, etc. in each dish. Why? Because we are looking at whole foods, the best foods on earth, remember, prepared with little fat and little salt, making these recipes the ideal companion to THE BEST DIET ON EARTH. One final, important point. *These meal plans and their recipes are the healthy way to weight loss, too.* Further discussion follows.

INTRODUCTION

Focus on Dinner

THE MEAL PLAN FOCUSES ON DINNER, because that's where the real challenge is. Every dinner for every day has been carefully planned with attention to taste (of course!), texture, and color. Yes, each dinner is color-coordinated and gives your eyes a treat. (Breakfast and lunch suggestions follow the dinner recipes.)

When you look at the meal plan, you will see that even a frozen, low-fat dinner can fit the bill. To make it a healthier choice, add an extra cup of cooked vegetables to the platter.

The Day After

GOURMET LUNCHES COME FROM WELL-PLANNED DINNERS. It's worth the cooking because you have great lunches the next day, lunches that will be the envy of your friends and co-workers. It's a happy day when "leftovers" are the makings for wonderful lunches. Top prize goes to "Meatloaf," and the runner-up is "Savory Salmon," both of which are delicious the day after.

Repetitious Breakfasts

WHO HAS TIME FOR BREAKFAST? Maybe you don't, but you know you have to eat it, that successful weight-losers eat it every day. Breakfast-eaters know the secret is in the repetition. Top prize here goes to Daily Eggs — four breakfasts in a row. Runner-up is Kashi cereals — tasty whole grain, high-fiber cereals that make filling and satisfying breakfasts.

Weight Loss

EACH DAY ON YOUR MEAL PLAN PROVIDES ABOUT 1500 CALORIES. This amount, plus regular exercise, translates into weight loss for most women. Men need more than 1500 calories per day, but they can still lose weight. How? By checking with a dietitian.

Products

THESE DESERVE SPECIAL MENTION because they are tops in taste and make your meal more satisfying, too.

☞ **Franklin Farms Veggie Burgers**

☞ **Lite English muffins** (not specific brand — has half the calories)

☞ **Manischewitz lite rye bread** (again — half the calories)

☞ **Taste of Thai or other hot sauce** ("Kick it up a notch," as the man says.)

☞ **Hummus** — a delicious spread that can easily take the place of mayo in a sandwich. It comes in all kinds of flavors: roasted garlic, sundried tomato and basil, roasted red peppers, and garden vegetable, to name a few.

☞ **Ajvar** — red pepper/eggplant purée, also known as "roasted red pepper sauce." It could well become your new ketchup!

☞ **Baked corn chips** (Tostitos, for example). Whole grain — and great dipped in ajvar.

DAY ONE

TERRIFIC TILAPIA

Four servings

1/2 cup thinly sliced scallions
1 tablespoon olive oil
2 teaspoons garlic, chopped
2 14.5-ounce cans of diced tomatoes, no salt added
1 1/2 teaspoons dried basil
1 pound tilapia, cut in 4 pieces

■ Sauté scallions in olive oil until tender about two minutes. Add garlic and cook until tender; add tomatoes and basil. Bring sauce to a light boil and then reduce heat to simmer.
■ Gently place fish in simmering sauce and poach until easily flaked with a fork, about 12 minutes.

BROCCOLI-CAULIFLOWER RIOT

Five 1/2-cup servings

1/2 cup celery, chopped
1/2 cup carrots, chopped
1/2 cup onion, chopped
1 package fresh broccoli and cauliflower flowers (4 cups raw)

■ Put all vegetables in medium saucepan and barely cover with water. Bring to a boil, then reduce heat and simmer, uncovered, until tender, about 10 minutes.

NOTES FOR THE COOK:
Tilapia is a wonderful mild, firm-textured white fish. Well worth a try. Serve over cooked pasta — any shape you prefer.

NOTES FOR THE COOK:
Give your broccoli and cauliflower a little extra attention; your family will love you for it.

UNBEATABLE BEET GREENS

About two 1/2-cup servings (depends on size of greens)

1 bunch of fresh red beets
Spray vegetable oil
2 cloves of garlic, minced
1/3 cup water

■ Cut the green leaves from the beet tops. Wash and cut up. Lightly spray nonstick pan and sauté garlic over low heat. Add beet leaves and let wilt. Add water, cover, and let steam for about 5 minutes, until tender.

GRANNY GRAPES WITH YOGURT

Six 1/2-cup servings

Spray vegetable oil
4 cups (about 1 1/2 pounds) red seedless grapes, the larger the
    better, washed and dried
3 cups fat-free yogurt, plain or vanilla

■ Preheat oven to 275°.
■ Lightly spray a nonstick baking sheet with sides. Spread grapes in a single layer. Bake for about 2 hours. The grapes go on a weight-loss diet in their sauna, so these will be smaller as well as wrinkled, but still soft and very juicy, when they are finished. Serve warm over 1/2-cup yogurt.

NOTES FOR THE COOK:
Fresh beets come with greens attached. DON'T THROW THEM AWAY! The greens are a tender flavorful, nutritious vegetable, a true "green".

NOTES FOR THE COOK:
If you have a sweet tooth, this dessert is for you. The baking intensifies the taste of the grapes, which get comfortably wrinkled (hence the name of this recipe) on their way to becoming tender, juicy raisins. Even though the cooking time is long, they require no attention. Talk about ambiance! A delicious dessert smell permeates the house.

DAY TWO

"MEATLOAF" ... OKAY, VEGETABLE AND TURKEY LOAF

Four servings

1 tablespoon olive oil
2 teaspoons garlic, chopped
1 cup celery, chopped
1 cup leeks, chopped
1 cup red pepper, chopped
1 1/2 cups mushrooms, chopped
1 pound ground turkey breast
1/4 cup egg substitute
1 slice whole wheat bread, processed in blender to
    make bread crumbs
Freshly ground pepper to taste

■ Preheat oven to 375°.
■ Heat olive oil in large, nonstick pan. Sauté all vegetables except mushrooms until beginning to brown, about 5 minutes. Add mushrooms and continue to sauté until all the vegetables are soft. Set aside.
■ Combine turkey, egg substitute, and bread crumbs in a large bowl. Add sautéed vegetables. Add pepper to taste. Transfer mixture to a loaf pan. Set pan in a baking dish and pour water into the baking dish until it is about half full. Bake the whole thing for 1 hour and 15 minutes.

NOTES FOR THE COOK:
Do you have fond memories of a meatloaf sandwich? This is an intriguing update of meatloaf—vegetable loaf with a wee bit of ground turkey.

NOTES FOR THE COOK:

A great mashed pota-to-plus combination. This is a real taste treat, a wonderful pairing of two shades of white. If you'd like to skip the potato peeling, be our guest! Scrub the skin well, and the result will be "smashed," rather than mashed, potatoes.

NOTES FOR THE COOK:

Is it a fruit? Is it a vegetable? Either way, it makes a nice, savory custard and proves that pumpkin custard doesn't absolutely have to be served in a pie shell. It doesn't even have to be sweet. By the way, this makes a nice brunch dish.

MASHED POTATOES AND CAULIFLOWER

Four 1/2-cup servings

2 medium red-skin potatoes, peeled and cubed
1 medium head cauliflower, florets only
1/4 cup Land O Lakes Fat Free Half & Half

■ Put potatoes and cauliflower in large saucepan, cover with water, and bring to a boil. Reduce heat and cook, covered, until vegetables are tender, about 20 minutes. Drain well and return to pot. Mash well. Add Half & Half and combine.

—————————————— ALTERNATIVE ——————————————

PUMPKIN PRIDE

Four 1/2-cup servings

3 tablespoons flour
3 tablespoons oil
1 cup fat-free milk
1/2 cup egg substitute
1 16-ounce can pumpkin, nothing added
Freshly ground pepper to taste
1 14.5-ounce can diced tomatoes, no salt added (Eden, for example), heated

■ Preheat oven to 350°.
■ Put oil and flour into small saucepan. Whisk together over low heat until well combined. Add milk; continue whisking until mixture is smooth and VERY thick. Remove from heat. Stir in egg substitute and pumpkin. Add pepper and stir again.
■ Put into 1-quart baking dish and put dish into a water bath (pan big enough to hold mold, with water added about half-way up the dish. This makes the Pumpkin Pride custard-y rather than dry). Put whole thing into oven. Bake until completely set, about one hour. Top with diced tomatoes.

RED AND GREEN

Eight 1/2-cup servings

Spray vegetable oil
1/4 cup sweet onion, chopped
4 large mushrooms, sliced (about 4 cups)
4 cups frozen whole green beans, thawed
1/4 cup sundried tomatoes in olive oil, drained and cut into strips
Freshly ground pepper to taste

■ Lightly spray large nonstick pan. Sauté onions until transparent. Add mushrooms and cook, stirring frequently, until nice and brown. Add beans, toss well, and continue to cook another few minutes, still stirring frequently, until beans are browned and tender. Mix in the sundried tomatoes and pepper.

NOTES FOR THE COOK:
Red and green — not just for Christmas anymore. Vegetables have to look good and be easy to fix. This recipes does the trick.

APPLE PIELESS

Four 1/2-cup servings

4 very large apples, peeled and sliced
2 heaping tablespoons apricot jam

■ Preheat oven to 350°.
■ Layer sliced apples in a pie dish. Spread with apricot jam. Bake 30 minutes or until tender and enjoy the apple pie smell, then pop under the broiler briefly, just to turn the apples golden brown.

NOTES FOR THE COOK:
"Pieless" because . . . there's no pie shell!

DAY THREE

LIMA DREAMS

Four 1/2-cup servings

2 10-ounce packages frozen lima beans
Spray vegetable oil
4 cloves garlic, chopped fine
Freshly ground pepper to taste
1 cup Land O Lakes Fat Free Half & Half

■ Cook lima beans according to directions on package. Lightly spray small skillet and sauté garlic until slightly browned. Drain beans and put into food processor. Add garlic, pepper, and Half & Half. Process until smooth.

GREENS AND WHEAT

Four 1/2-cup servings

Spray vegetable oil
2 medium onions, chopped
3 cloves garlic, chopped fine
Small head escarole, washed and coarsely chopped
2 tablespoons lemon juice
2 cups water
1 cup bulgar wheat
Freshly ground pepper to taste

■ Lightly spray large nonstick skillet. Sauté onions and garlic until onions are transparent. Add escarole and lemon juice and cook, covered, until greens start to wilt. (If your skillet has no lid, use foil instead.) Add water and bulgar, stir, and cover again. Cook until liquid is absorbed, about 15 minutes. Add pepper.

NOTES FOR THE COOK: This is a personal favorite. What a great recipe! Not only delicious, but a truly gorgeous green. It is equally tasty served hot or at room temperature. Use leftovers as a wonderful sandwich spread, or try on whole grain crackers.

NOTES FOR THE COOK: It's not unusual to pair escarole with beans ("scarola e fagioli," in Italy) and here we're combining escarole and bulgar. Sorry, we don't know the Italian for bulgar, but we do know it's delicious.

—————————— ALTERNATIVE ——————————

QUINOA WOW

Six 1/2-cup servings

1/2 cup quinoa
1 cup water
Spray vegetable oil
1 clove garlic, chopped fine
1/2 cup chopped onion
1/2 cup frozen yellow corn kernels
1 small-ish zucchini, chopped
1 14.5-ounce can diced tomatoes, no salt added
1 10-ounce package frozen peas, thawed
4 fresh basil leaves, chopped
Freshly ground pepper to taste

■ Put quinoa into a strainer and rinse under running water. Allow to drain. Transfer to saucepan, add water, and simmer, covered, until water is absorbed and quinoa is nice and fluffy, about 15 minutes.

■ Meanwhile, lightly spray a nonstick skillet with oil and sauté the onions and garlic until the onions are transparent. Add zucchini and cook until lightly browned. Stir in tomatoes, corn, peas, and basil and continue cooking until vegetables are tender, which will be just a very few minutes.

■ Fluff up the quinoa-corn mixture and combine with the vegetables.

NOTES FOR THE COOK:
One of our mothers introduced us to this wonderful grain-like food. We've been saying all along that moms know best. Pronounced "KEEN-wa," when cooked, each tiny piece becomes translucent and has a lovely ring inside. Quite special.

NOTES FOR THE COOK:

Hm-m-m-m. What is "zest"? If you thought it had something to do with enthusiasm, not food, you were half right. In this sense, it applies to citrus fruit, and is the thin, outer part of the rind. You can scrape or grate the fruit to get the zest. You can also use a zester. (There does seem to be a tool for everything, doesn't there?) Simple enough is a vegetable peeler. You'll have pieces that you can cut into strips and then chop coarsely.

ZESTY ORANGE DESSERT

Two servings (easily doubled; allow 1 orange per serving)

1 tablespoon chopped lemon zest (from one of the oranges)
2 teaspoons Grand Marnier liqueur
1/4 cup orange juice
1/2 teaspoon lemon juice
2 medium navel oranges

■ Put zest into small saucepan with water to cover. Bring to a boil, then drain. Combine with liqueur, orange juice, and lemon juice. Peel and slice oranges. There shouldn't be any seeds, but if there are, remove them. Arrange orange slices prettily on two plates. Drizzle with orange mixture.

DAY FOUR

MEAL IN A BOWL

Eight 1-cup servings

1-1/2 pounds boneless, skinless chicken breasts
Dried herb mixture
Heavy aluminum foil large enough to make envelope around
    chicken
1 48-ounce can chicken broth, fat free and low sodium
1 14.5-ounce can chicken broth, ditto
1/2 cup barley
2 teaspoons dried basil
1 teaspoon thyme
2 16-ounce packages frozen corn kernels, thawed, divided
1 cup water
1 cup celery, chopped
1 cup carrots, chopped
1/2 cup sliced scallions
Freshly ground pepper to taste

■ Preheat oven to 400°.
■ Rinse chicken breasts in cold water; pat dry with paper towel. Lay in single layer on foil and sprinkle with dried herb mixture. Seal foil, place in baking dish, and bake for 45 minutes.
■ Meanwhile, bring broth to a boil. Add barley, basil, and thyme, reduce heat, and simmer, covered, for 30 minutes.
■ Into food processor, put one package corn and I cup water. Purée.
■ When soup has finished simmering, add puréed corn, chopped celery, and carrots, scallions, and other package of corn. Cook over low heat for 15 minutes. Season with pepper.
■ When chicken is cooked and cool enough to handle, cut into bite-size pieces and put them, along with the juice in the foil, into the soup. Serve piping hot.

NOTES FOR THE COOK:
This has a lot of ingredients, but don't be fooled. It's very, very easy, and you end up with a delicious thick, hearty soup — with only one pot to clean!

**NOTES FOR
THE COOK:**

Fruit and salad are
wonderful, healthy
combinations, and
you'll find you need
less dressing when
you use fruit.
Strawberries work
well, and you might
also try melon in
season. Apples are
good all year long.

STRAWBERRY
AND SPINACH SALAD

Four servings

2 tablespoons canola oil
2 tablespoons cider vinegar
1 teaspoon dried onions
1 teaspoon sugar
1 pint fresh strawberries, stems removed and sliced
1 6-ounce bag prewashed baby spinach

■ Make dressing first, so the flavors have a chance to blend.
■ Combine oil, vinegar, dried onions, and sugar in a small jar, shake
well, and set aside.
■ Combine spinach and strawberries. Add dressing, let salad sit for
a few minutes, then serve.

DAY FIVE

SHRIMP WITH TOMATOES

Four 1-cup servings

1/4 cup lemon juice
2 teaspoons olive oil
2 cloves garlic, crushed
1 pound medium fresh shrimp, peeled (about 32 shrimp)
1 28-ounce can crushed tomatoes
Freshly ground pepper to taste

■ Combine lemon juice, olive oil, and garlic in a small bowl. Toss with shrimp. Cover with plastic wrap. Allow to marinate several hours in the refrigerator. (If you decide late in the day to make this, set bowl on counter for 1/2 hour before cooking.)

■ Remove shrimp from marinade and add liquid to tomatoes. Heat tomato mixture in a medium saucepan. While it is heating, cook shrimp by stir-frying in a well-heated nonstick skillet for about 3 minutes or so. Allow to brown slightly. Add to tomatoes and season with pepper.

NOTES FOR THE COOK:
Shrimp is very low in fat and, in moderate amounts, good for a healthy diet. Serving the shrimp and tomatoes with Eggplant Rice is wonderful.

**NOTES FOR
THE COOK:**
You'll certainly want
to be experimenting
with new flavors and
tastes, and this recipe
will help you do just
that. It's a truly
interesting as well as
delicious
combination. While
you're at it, why not
use brown rice? It has
a well-earned
reputation for being
particularly good for
you. If you think of
brown rice as being
sticky or chewy, try
Uncle Ben's Original
Brown Rice. It is
neither of the above,
and it tastes very, very
good.

EGGPLANT RICE

Six 1/2-cup servings

Spray vegetable oil
1 medium eggplant, unpeeled and cubed
1/2 cup onion, chopped
2 cloves garlic, chopped fine
1 cup rice, white or brown (if you go brown, find one that takes
    about 30 minutes to cook)
1 14.5-ounce can low-sodium fat-free chicken broth

■ Spray medium saucepan lightly with oil. Add eggplant and cook over high heat, stirring frequently, until slightly browned. Reduce heat. Add onion and garlic, stirring until onion is soft. Add rice, tossing it with eggplant, and then stir well, browning the rice a bit. Pour in broth, bring to boil, then reduce heat. Cook covered until liquid is absorbed, about 20-25 minutes, maybe another 10 minutes for longer-cooking brown rice.

DAY SIX

"Fried" Chicken
Four servings

2 slices whole wheat bread, processed in blender to make
    bread crumbs
1/2 teaspoon marjoram
1/2 teaspoon paprika
1/4 cup grated Parmesan or soy parmesan cheese
1 teaspoon garlic powder
1/4 teaspoon freshly ground pepper
1 pound boneless, skinless chicken breasts, each cut into 5 strips
1/2 cup of buttermilk

■ Preheat oven to 350°.
■ Mix bread crumbs with marjoram, paprika, Parmesan, pepper, and garlic powder. Dip chicken strips in buttermilk. Roll in bread-crumb mixture. Place on wire rack, set on baking sheet, and bake for 40 minutes, until golden brown.

NOTES FOR THE COOK:
By the way, it's not fried. This is a KFC alternative, a marvelous meal. It looks like it's hard to make because of the number of ingredients, but it isn't. Serve over Mango Slaw, the following recipe.

Mango Slaw

Six 1-cup servings

2 tablespoons honey
2 tablespoons canola oil
3 tablespoons lime juice
Freshly ground pepper to taste
3 cups shredded red cabbage
2 cups shredded savory cabbage
1 cup peeled, julienned carrots
1 ripe mango, peeled and seeded, cut in 1/2-inch pieces (or frozen
    pieces, thawed)

■ In a small bowl, mix together honey, canola oil, lime juice, and pepper. In a large bowl, place red and savoy cabbages and carrots. Toss to mix well. Add honey-lime mixture and mango, tossing gently. Arrange cabbage mixture on platter with chicken on top.

--------------------- **ALTERNATIVE** ---------------------
(Check the Meal Plan for Day Six. This substitutes
for Chicken and Mango Slaw, and for your corn-on-the-cob):

LAGOON CHICKEN SALAD
Four servings

4 halves boneless, skinless chicken breasts (about 4 ounces each)
1 1/2 cups unsweetened apple juice
3 cups cooked wild rice, prepared according to package directions
1 1/2 cups seedless green grapes, halved
1 cup unpeeled apple, chopped
1/2 cup celery, chopped
3/4 cup slivered almonds, divided
1/2 cup water chestnuts, chopped
Yogurt-Mustard Dressing (recipe follows)
Spinach leaves

■ Rinse chicken breasts in cold water; pat dry with paper towel.
Place chicken in deep saucepan. Add apple juice and cook over
medium heat about 15 minutes, or until fork can be easily inserted.
Remove chicken from pan and allow chicken to cool.
■ Dice chicken and gently toss with wild rice, grapes, apple, celery,
1/2 cup of the slivered almonds, and water chestnuts. Add dressing
and toss lightly. Cover and chill about 30 minutes to blend flavors.
■ To serve, place spinach leaves on platter; spoon on chicken mixture and sprinkle with remaining almonds.

**National Chicken
Cooking Contest
Recipe**

YOGURT-MUSTARD DRESSING
Makes 1 cup

1 cup fat-free plain yogurt
1 tablespoon Dijon mustard
Freshly ground pepper to taste

■ Combine well in small bowl.

NOTES FOR THE COOK:
We all want to end our meal with a dessert. Something warm, with a delicious smell, and a wonderful sweet taste. Roasted Pineapple is all three.

ROASTED PINEAPPLE SLICES
About four servings

Spray cooking oil
Whole pineapple, unpeeled, washed and sliced into rounds
2 tablespoons apricot jam

■ Preheat oven to 400°.
■ Spray cookie sheet with nonstick spray. Place pineapple slices on tray. Spread with apricot jam. Cook for 15 minutes.

DAY SEVEN

VEGETARIAN-FOR-BEGINNERS PIE

Four servings

3/4 cup brown rice (try Uncle Ben's instant)
1 large onion, chopped
1 tablespoon olive oil
1/2 cup egg substitute
1 cup fat-free milk
1 cup canned pink beans, no salt added, drained and rinsed
2 ounces Cabot low-fat cheddar cheese, grated
1 teaspoon dried tarragon
1 teaspoon Worcestershire sauce
Spray cooking oil

■ Preheat oven to 325°.

■ Cook rice according to package directions. Sauté onion in olive oil. Mix egg substitute and milk in a large bowl, add cooked rice, beans, sautéed onions, cheese, tarragon, and Worcestershire sauce. Turn mixture into a 9 X 9 glass dish that has been lightly sprayed with oil. Place baking dish in a larger pan and pour water between the pans. Bake for 1 hour or until top of custard is firm and edges are golden brown. Let sit 10 minutes before serving.

NOTES FOR THE COOK:

All sorts of great items are hanging out in the produce section, like plastic bags of fresh broccoli "florets" (just those little green tops), all washed and ready to go.

BROCCOLI TO LIVE FOR

Four 1/2-cup servings

Spray vegetable oil
2 garlic cloves, chopped
1 12-ounce package fresh broccoli florets
1 cup white wine (try a dry wine, but if you prefer a sweeter one, that's fine)
Freshly ground pepper to taste

■ Lightly spray a nonstick saucepan and brown the garlic. Add broccoli and toss to distribute the garlic a bit, and then add the wine. Cover pan and simmer for about 10 minutes (you can adjust the time, depending on how crisp or soft you like your broccoli); remove broccoli to serving platter using slotted spoon. Turn up heat on pan and boil wine and garlic until most of the liquid has evaporated. This will concentrate the flavors while you concentrate on something else. But don't overdo it — the liquid will quickly boil away. Pour over broccoli. Season with pepper.

ADVENTUROUS SALAD

Make enough so that each serving is 2-3 cups

1 or more 6-ounce (approximately) packages cut-up romaine lettuce
1 small head radicchio
1 or more 6-ounce (approximately) packages baby spinach leaves
Chives
Sundried tomatoes
Carrot slivers
Broccoli slaw
Broccoli sprouts
Marinated red peppers (comes in a jar)
Red beets (canned)
For additional taste and pleasure, try one or more of the following
    "blend-ins."
Walnuts
Apple slices
Mandarin orange slices
Melon, cut up
Craisins
Banana slices
Sunflower seeds
Avocado

■ Mix everything together and toss lightly with your favorite dressing. If you don't have a favorite, try "Our Favorite Oil and Vinegar Dressing."

NOTES FOR THE COOK:
Salad can be more than iceberg lettuce, winter tomatoes, and cucumbers, which can be pretty boring. This is the time to be inspired. Be bold and adventurous, putting some things into your salad that you might not have thought of. Pick from this list! Opportunity is knocking, so this is your chance!

OUR FAVORITE OIL AND VINEGAR DRESSING

Makes 6 tablespoons

1/4 cup olive oil
1/8 cup balsamic or red wine vinegar
1 teaspoon Dijon mustard
Freshly ground pepper to taste

◼ Combine all ingredients in a small jar. Shake well.

STRAWBERRIES TARTAR

Makes about 2 cups

2 cups strawberries, the riper the better, washed and hulled (stems
    and cores removed)
1/8 teaspoon black pepper
1 1/2 teaspoons balsamic vinegar

◼ Put berries in large bowl. Chop completely, using a knife or a chopping blade. Berries should be in tiny little pieces and extremely juicy when you are finished. Stir in pepper and vinegar.

NOTES FOR THE COOK:

A seemingly strange combination, but it works. Put on top of a whole grain waffle as a wonderful adults-only topping. Use plenty- it's fruit! Today, put it on your salad!

DAY EIGHT

CAREFREE FLOUNDER

Four servings

1 pound fresh flounder fillets
4 teaspoons Dijon mustard
2 tablespoons lemon juice
1/3 cup white wine

■ Preheat oven to 350°.
■ Lay the flounder in a single layer in a baking dish. Spread with mustard. Pour lemon juice and wine over all, and bake for 20 minutes. (If this strikes you as being just a little too simple, cut up a carrot, a medium tomato, and half a small onion. Put on top of fish before you put it in the oven.)

VEGETABLE GARDEN

Four 1/2-cup servings

1/4 cup canned vegetable broth
1 medium sweet white onion, sliced
6 large fresh mushrooms, sliced
1 yellow pepper, cored, seeded and cut up
1 medium zucchini, cubed
Mrs. Dash Seasoning Blend
4 fresh plum tomatoes, coarsely chopped

■ Put broth and onion in a large, nonstick skillet. Cover and simmer until onion is soft. Add mushrooms, pepper, and zucchini. Sprinkle with Mrs. Dash. Stir frequently while vegetables cook, until liquid evaporates and they start to brown, about 10-15 minutes. Add tomatoes and (again) stir frequently as they cook into the vegetables.

NOTES FOR THE COOK: The most time-consuming part of this recipe is unwrapping the fish.

NOTES FOR THE COOK: Browning vegetables without fat shows you have reached the heights of excellence in cooking for health. We both have husbands who love to eat. If the food didn't taste good, they wouldn't eat it. And they love this.

**NOTES FOR
THE COOK:**
Warm, cozy, and
altogether perfect for
enjoying by the fire.

HEARTHSIDE FRUIT

Four 1/2-cup servings

1 8 1/4-ounce can pears in juice
1 8 1/4-ounce can peaches in juice
1 cup dried fruit bits (Sun-Maid, for example)
2 teaspoons lemon juice
1 teaspoon vanilla extract

■ Empty cans of pears and peaches, juice and all, into small saucepan. Add dried fruit and lemon juice. Combine and heat through. Remove from heat and stir in vanilla extract.

DAY NINE

HEARTY MOROCCAN CHICKEN
Six servings

6 chicken leg quarters, skinned
1 tablespoon olive oil
1 medium onion, cut in chunks
4 cloves garlic, minced
1 tablespoon minced fresh ginger
2 carrots, peeled and cut in chunks
1 cup no-salt-added canned chickpeas, rinsed and drained
1/2 cup golden raisins
2 sticks cinnamon
1 1/2 teaspoons cumin
1/2 teaspoon turmeric
5 cups water
2 zucchini, cut in chunks
2 cups prepared couscous, whole wheat

■ Rinse chicken in cold water; pat dry with paper towel. Put olive oil into large, nonstick skillet and place over high heat. Add chicken and cook about 10 minutes, turning to brown on all sides. Stir in onion, garlic, ginger, carrots, chickpeas, raisins, cinnamon, cumin, turmeric, and water. Bring to a simmer, reduce heat, and cook about 20 minutes. Stir in zucchini and cook an additional 10 minutes. Remove cinnamon sticks. Serve in large bowls over couscous.

National Chicken Cooking Contest Recipe

NOTES FOR THE COOK: DASH goes exotic and delicious. Convenient, too. Leg quarters come already skinned and frozen!

NOTES FOR THE COOK:

Escarole — pronounced "Es-ka-roll" — looks like a mini-romaine, only smoother, and the leaves are heavier. It's great in salad, mixed with other greens, and wonderful in soup, too.

SASSY ESCAROLE

Four 1/2-cup servings

2 small-to-medium heads escarole
1 tablespoon olive oil
1 medium onion, chopped
Freshly ground pepper to taste

■ Cut off the bottom couple of inches of the escarole heads, which will separate the leaves and remove the tougher ends. Wash well and cut up coarsely. (There will seem to be an awful lot of it, but it shrinks as it cooks.)

■ In a big pot, the kind you might use to make pasta or soup, put the olive oil. Heat it a bit and add the onion. Cook until transparent, stirring occasionally. Add the escarole, still wet from being washed. Cover and cook over medium heat (it will steam from the water on the leaves) until tender and much reduced, about 10-15 minutes. Season with pepper.

NOTES FOR THE COOK:

If you've never tasted roasted red beets, now's your chance. A cousin told us the secret of wrapping the raw beats in foil and then cooking them in the oven. Easy to peel when they're done. Just rub with a paper towel and the skin comes right off. Don't worry if your hands turn red. The color will wash off.

ROASTED RED BEET SALAD

Four 1-cup servings

4 large fresh red beets
1/4 cup orange juice
1 1/2 teaspoons honey
1 1/2 teaspoons balsamic vinegar
1 teaspoon olive oil
1 teaspoon Dijon mustard
1 tablespoon "snipped" fresh chives (use scissors to cut them up)
1 package baby spinach leaves (approximately 6 ounces)

■ Preheat oven to 350°.
■ Wrap beets in foil. Bake until tender, about 1 1/4 hours. Meanwhile, make dressing by whisking together the juice, honey, vinegar, and oil. When beets are cooked, unless you have asbestos hands, allow to cool enough so you can handle them. When they're cool, cut off stem end and peel — very easy. Slice beets and toss with dressing. Sprinkle with chives and toss again. Serve on spinach leaves.

DAY TEN

SAVORY SALMON

Four servings

1 pound fresh salmon fillet (ask to have any large bones removed)
Heavy aluminum foil to make a tray for fish
2 tablespoons soy sauce
2 tablespoons honey

■ Place salmon skin side down on an aluminum foil bed with sides and lay on a baking sheet. Blend soy sauce and honey; coat salmon with mixture. Broil in upper part of oven, basting very frequently. The more you baste the more golden brown the salmon will be. Broil for about 15 minutes (longer if you prefer it better done), or until fish is flaky.

——————— ALTERNATIVE ———————

SALMON COOKED IN FOIL

Four servings

1 pound fresh salmon fillet (ask to have any large bones removed)
1 scallion, chopped
4 pieces sun-dried tomatoes that come marinated in olive oil;
    drained well and blotted with paper towels, then snipped in strips
1 tablespoon fresh tarragon (or other herb of your choice),
    snipped in small pieces
1/4 cup dry white wine
Freshly ground pepper to taste
Heavy aluminum foil, large enough to make an envelope around
    fish

■ Preheat oven to 450°.
■ Lay salmon on foil. Sprinkle with scallion, sun-dried tomatoes, and tarragon (or other herb). Grind fresh pepper over all. Carefully pour wine over fish, seal aluminum pouch, lay in ovenproof dish, and bake for 25 minutes.

NOTES FOR THE COOK:
This is a great way to make salmon if you are a first-timer. You end up with a beautiful, glazed fish fillet. By the way — buy extra, so you'll have leftovers to make "The Best Salmon Salad" (recipe later).

NOTES FOR THE COOK:
Cooking in foil holds in juices and has the added advantage of leaving you with a pan that needs little or no scrubbing.

NOTES FOR
THE COOK:
After you've tried this
recipe, experiment
with other
potato/vegetable
combinations.
Grandkids will love it.

MASHED MADNESS: POTATOES, SWEET POTATOES, AND CARROTS

Four 1/2-cup servings

2 medium boiling potatoes, peeled and cut up
2 medium sweet potatoes, ditto
1 cup carrots, ditto
1/4 cup Land O Lakes Fat Free Half & Half
1/2 teaspoon dried thyme leaves
Freshly ground pepper to taste

■ Put potatoes and carrots into medium saucepan, cover with water, and bring to a boil. Reduce heat, cover pot, and simmer until vegetables are tender, about 30 minutes. Drain well, then mash until smooth. Add Half & Half, whipping into potato-carrot mixture.

——————————— ALTERNATIVE ———————————

FRUITY SWEET POTATOES

Four 1/2-cup servings

2 very large sweet potatoes (about 2 lbs. total), unpeeled and cut up
1 cup dried pitted prunes, quartered
1/2 cup water
1 cup canned pineapple pieces in juice, no sugar added, drained

■ Preheat oven to 350°.
■ Put potato pieces into medium saucepan, cover generously with water, and bring to a boil. Reduce heat and cook covered until very soft, about 35-40 minutes.
■ Meanwhile, simmer prunes in water for 5 minutes. Do not drain. When potatoes are tender, drain them and remove skin, which will peel off easily. Mash well. Stir in pineapple and prunes. Spoon into baking dish for about 20 minutes, or until heated through.

NOTES FOR
THE COOK:
A perfect
Thanksgiving dish,
but good all year. Can
be prepared ahead
and refrigerated, but
allow to come to room
temperature before
heating.

DAY ELEVEN

Sweet 'n Sour Pork Loins

Four servings

3 cloves of garlic, split in half
1 tablespoon olive oil
1 pound pork tenderloins
1 large onion, sliced
2 tablespoons brown sugar
1/3 cup raisins
1/4 cup balsamic vinegar
1 14-ounce can tomato sauce, no salt added
2 teaspoons hot sauce (maybe "A Taste of Thai Garlic Chili Pepper
   Sauce")

■ Preheat oven to 350°.

■ In a large, nonstick pan, sauté garlic in olive oil over medium heat until beginning to turn color. Add pork loins and sauté on high heat until golden brown. Place loins and garlic in a covered baking dish.

■ Sauté onion in same pan on high heat, stirring constantly until transparent. Add brown sugar and keep stirring until brown sugar is bubbly. Mix in raisins, balsamic vinegar, tomato sauce, and hot sauce. Simmer for five minutes. Pour onion/raisin sauce mixture over chops. Bake for 1 hour and 15 minutes.

NOTES FOR THE COOK:
This is really wonderful served over brown rice.

————————— ALTERNATIVE —————————

Sweet 'n Sour Pork Loins II

Four servings

1 pound pork tenderloins
1 tablespoon olive oil
1 large onion, sliced
2 tablespoons brown sugar
1/3 cup craisins
3/4 cup orange juice
1/4 teaspoon cinnamon
1/4 teaspoon ginger

■ Preheat oven to 350°.
■ In a large nonstick pan, sauté pork in olive oil over high heat until golden brown. Place in a baking dish and cover.
■ Sauté onions in same pan over high heat, stirring constantly until transparent. Add brown sugar and stir constantly until brown sugar is bubbly. Mix in craisins, orange juice, cinnamon, and ginger. Pour onion/craisin sauce mixture over pork. Bake for 1 hour and 15 minutes.

NOTES FOR THE COOK:

"There's always another way," our mothers used to tell us when we was trying to figure things out. We admit that pork chops were not the subject of the conversation. Nevertheless, the sentiment certainly applies. Like the other pork loins, these are delicious served over brown rice.

GREENS AND CHERRIES

Six 1/2-cup servings

1 tablespoon canola oil
3 cups sliced onion (a sweet variety, like Vidalia, if available)
3 large bunches fresh greens such as collard, stemmed if necessary, and coarsely chopped (about 12 cups)
1/4 teaspoon salt
1 cup canned unsweetened sour cherries, drained

■ Heat the oil in a large, deep skillet or Dutch oven. Add the onion and sauté over high heat for about 5 minutes. Turn the heat to medium/high and, stirring frequently, let the onion cook until slightly caramelized (about 5 more minutes).

■ Begin adding the greens in batches (as much as will fit), sprinkling a tiny bit of the salt with each addition. Stir and cover between additions, letting the greens cook down for about 2 minutes each time to make room for the next batch.

■ When all the greens are added and have cooked to tender (about 20 minutes for collards), stir in the cherries and cook for just about 5 minutes longer. Transfer to a platter. Serve hot or warm, being sure to include some of the delicious cooking juices with each serving.

■ Note that the time it takes for a green to become tender will depend on the type and "youthfulness" of the greens. Tender young greens can be cooked in a matter of minutes.

NOTES FOR THE COOK:
Not to be confused with cherry pie filling, these sour cherries pair nicely with greens, in a combination that is delicious and very pretty besides. If you're from cherry-picking country, and one of us is, you know what it means to have a fondness for cherries.

**NOTES FOR
THE COOK:**
We come from a long
line of recipe clippers.
Mom clipped this
years ago and then
made it her way. We
loved it, and we pass it
on to you.

TANGY TURNIPS

Four 1/2-cup servings

3 small-to-medium turnips, peeled and sliced (about 4 cups)
1 tablespoon canola oil
2 teaspoons cornstarch
1 cup low-sodium fat-free chicken broth, divided in half
3 scallions, sliced
1 1/2 cups watercress, large stems removed
1 teaspoon garlic, chopped
1 teaspoon ground ginger
1 teaspoon brown sugar

■ Soak turnips in ice water for about 15 minutes, then pat dry. Put oil in large, nonstick skillet, heat, and cook turnips over medium heat, stirring frequently. Meanwhile, dissolve cornstarch in 1/2 cup chicken broth. When turnips have cooked for 5 minutes, reduce heat to low and add cornstarch mixture. It will sizzle and sort of start to disappear, but don't worry. That's what you're saving the rest of the chicken broth for, and we'll get to that in a minute.
■ Stir in the scallions, watercress, garlic, ginger, and brown sugar. Slowly stir in other 1/2 cup of chicken broth. If turnips are not tender enough for you at this point, continue to cook them gently, stirring frequently, until they are just the way you want them.

DAY TWELVE

YIN YANG SOUP

Four 1-cup servings

1 medium cantaloupe, rind and seeds removed, and cut up
1 medium honeydew melon, ditto
1 red bell pepper, seeded and diced
2 tablespoons fresh basil, finely chopped
Juice of one lime
2 tablespoons fresh mint, finely chopped

■ Purée each melon separately, pour each purée into a pitcher, and refrigerate. When you are ready to serve, stir the soups and pour them AT EXACTLY THE SAME TIME into chilled soup plates. Garnish cantaloupe purée with red pepper and basil, and honeydew purée with lime juice and mint.

───────────────────

THREE-IN-ONE: Rice, Beans, and Spinach

Four 1/2-cup servings

Spray vegetable oil
1 medium onion, chopped
1 cup canned beans (white or navy), no salt added, rinsed and
    drained
1/2 cup Uncle Ben's Brown Rice (for other brown rice, allow a little
    more cooking time
1 14.5-ounce can low-sodium fat-free chicken broth
1 10-ounce package frozen chopped spinach, thawed
Freshly ground pepper to taste

■ Lightly spray large, nonstick skillet. Brown onion slightly. Reduce heat and add rice, tossing briefly. Add broth, cover, and cook for 15 minutes. Stir in spinach and beans; cook another 15-20 minutes, until liquid is absorbed and rice is tender. Season with pepper.

NOTES FOR THE COOK:
Fruit soups are very popular these days. This one would be especially nice at a brunch, too, being glorious to look at and truly delectable to eat.

NOTES FOR THE COOK:
Here is a grain (rice), and legume (beans), and a vegetable (spinach), all working for you at once. If you are new to the beans game, this is for you.

**NOTES FOR
THE COOK:**

"Braising" means
cooking with a small
amount of liquid. The
kale remains beautiful
and green. Leafy
greens are like kittens
— tender and inviting
when they are small,
but tougher and a
little hard to
approach when they
are older. And they
get old really, really
quickly.

BRAISED KALE
WITH WHITE BEANS

Four 1/2-cup servings

Spray vegetable oil
I medium onion, chopped
1 bunch fresh kale, washed, with stems cut off and coarsely
    chopped
2 packages Herb-ox Chicken Bouillon, very low sodium, dissolved
    in 1 1/2 cups boiling water, divided
1 15-ounce can white or navy beans, no salt added, rinsed and
    drained
Freshly ground pepper to taste

■ Lightly spray large, nonstick skillet with oil, add chopped onion
and brown slightly, stirring frequently. Add kale, pour half the broth
(3/4 cup) over it, and cook uncovered over medium heat, stirring
frequently. When liquid evaporates, add rest of broth, reduce heat,
and continue cooking (and stirring) until kale is tender, about 10
minutes in all. (If liquid evaporates before kale is as tender as you
would like, add another 1/4 cup of water.) Toss with beans, heat
through, and season with pepper.

QUICKIE EGGPLANT PLUS

Four 1/2-cup servings

Spray vegetable oil
1 large sweet onion, sliced
2 cloves garlic, chopped fine
4 small-ish zucchini, cubed
1 medium eggplant, peeled and cubed
1 teaspoon dried oregano
Freshly ground pepper
6 plum tomatoes, sliced

■ Preheat oven to 375°.
■ Lightly spray large, nonstick, ovenproof skillet. Sauté onion and garlic until onion is transparent. Add zucchini and eggplant and cook over medium heat, stirring frequently, until vegetables are just beginning to get soft, which will take less than 5 minutes. Sir in oregano and pepper. Cover with tomato slices and bake until tomatoes are soft and vegetables are tender, 15-20 minutes.

NOTES FOR THE COOK:
This is ratatouille-like, so make extra, because it's delicious in a sandwich. Come home from work and need something to tide you over until dinner? Try this with a few whole grain crackers.

DAY THIRTEEN

UNLIKELY CHICKEN

Four servings

4 halves boneless and skinless chicken breast (about 4 ounces each)
1/3 cup nonfat plain yogurt
1/3 cup apricot or raspberry all-fruit preserves
1 tablespoon Dijon mustard

■ Preheat oven to 350°.
■ Rinse chicken breasts in cold water; pat dry with paper towel. Place in a small, shallow baking dish in a single layer. Combine yogurt, preserves, and mustard (we know, we know, but trust us), spread mixture over the chicken breasts, and bake uncovered for 45 minutes.

VEGETABLES OF SPRING

Six 1/2-cup servings

8 small red-skinned potatoes, cubed
1 14.5-ounce can low-sodium fat-free chicken broth
1/2 cup white wine (dry or sweet, your choice)
1 10-ounce package frozen lima beans, thawed
12 asparagus spears cut up
1 10-ounce package frozen peas, thawed
1 medium tomato, chopped

■ Put potatoes and broth into medium saucepan, bring to a boil, reduce heat, and cook, covered, for several minutes, just until potatoes start to get soft. Add wine, lima beans, and asparagus. Do not cover. Continue cooking until vegetables are tender, about 10 minutes in all. Turn off heat. Add peas and tomatoes and toss until heated through.

NOTES FOR THE COOK:
The combination of ingredients gives this dish its name. They look rather — ahem — strange. Just goes to show that you can't always judge a recipe by reading it! Good cold, too.

NOTES FOR THE COOK:
We have experienced many springs in our lives. We bring this really pretty and tasty dish so that you too may have many springs. It is slightly soupy, so don't be surprised. That's part of the charm.

ROMANTIC GLAZED STRAWBERRIES

Four servings

1/4 cup currant jelly, melted
12 big, beautiful, long-stemmed strawberries, washed and chilled
Serving plate, chilled in the refrigerator

■ Put jelly into a small bowl and dip each strawberry into it, twirling it gently to coat. Immediately place on chilled plate. Return berries to refrigerator until ready to serve.

NOTES FOR THE COOK:
It's nice when something beautiful and delicious is also incredibly easy to make.

DAY FOURTEEN

Salmon Croquettes
Four servings

2 6-ounce cans salmon
1 small onion, chopped
2 stalks celery, chopped
1/4 red pepper, chopped
1/4 cup egg substitute
2 heaping tablespoons ajvar (red pepper spread) — optional
1/4 cup seasoned breadcrumbs
Spray vegetable oil

■ Preheat oven to 300°.
■ Mix together everything but cooking oil and breadcrumbs and form into twelve small patties. Coat with breadcrumbs. Spray nonstick pan and "fry" the patties in batches, four at a time, turning once, and spraying between batches. Cook until golden brown on both sides.
■ Place on baking sheet and bake for ten minutes.

SUCCOTASH BASH
Four 1/2-cup servings

Spray vegetable oil
1 scallion, chopped, including green
1 cup canned low-sodium fat-free chicken broth
1 teaspoon dried tarragon
1 16-ounce package frozen succotash
1 cup grape tomato halves
Freshly ground pepper to taste

■ Lightly spray nonstick skillet. Sauté scallion until lightly browned. Add broth, tarragon, and succotash. Cook until vegetables have nearly reached desired tenderness, about 5-7 minutes. Add tomatoes and toss. Heat through.

NOTES FOR THE COOK:
The combination of colors in this hearty dish is, surprisingly, quite spectacular.

And so, working from the start of the day, we come to -

BREAKFAST

DAILY EGGS
Four servings

Spray vegetable oil
1 8-ounce container egg substitute (equivalent to 4 eggs)
2 heaping tablespoons ajvar
Breakfast Veggies (recipe follows)

■ Lightly spray nonstick pan. Combine next three ingredients and scramble. One quarter of the eggs makes a good breakfast, so store remainder in refrigerator for breakfast the next three days. Prep is a snap! Just reheat in microwave until eggs are as hot as you like.

BREAKFAST VEGGIES
Makes about 1 cup

Spray vegetable oil
1 small onion, chopped
1 green or red pepper, chopped
8-ounce package of sliced mushrooms
1 small zucchini, sliced
(Any leftover cooked broccoli? Chop and add!)

■ Lightly spray nonstick pan and sauté onion until transparent. Add green pepper, mushrooms, and zucchini and continue cooking until slightly crunchy- tender.

**NOTES FOR
THE COOK:**

No time for breakfast?
No excuses. Ready in a
jiffy — drink it and
you're on your way.

FAST AND FRUITY BREAKFAST
Makes 2 cups

1/2 cup orange juice
4 whole frozen strawberries
1 very ripe banana (over-ripe is okay), cut up
1 cup fat-free yogurt, any flavor (try vanilla or a berry flavor)

■ Put all into blender and purée until smooth.

**NOTES FOR
THE COOK:**

A nice change of pace,
this is a tasty two-fer
that combines fruit
and low-fat (in this
case, fat-free) dairy.
The dried fruit bits
expand and become
tender and flavorful.
By the way — when the
pudding is cooling, a
skin forms over the
top when it is exposed
to the air. If you don't
like that, lay a piece of
plastic wrap directly
on the pudding when
you set it out to cool.

FRUIT-FILLED RICE PUDDING
Five 1/2-cup servings

5 1/2 cups fat-free milk
1/2 cup sugar
2 teaspoons vanilla extract
3/4 cup rice
3/4 cup Sun-Maid Fruit Bits (these are dried)
Sprig of fresh mint

■ Put the milk, sugar, and vanilla into a saucepan. Bring to a boil, stir in the rice, reduce heat, and cook, covered, over low heat for 45 minutes. The rice will be soft and the mixture will be soupy, which is what you want. It will firm up as it cools.
■ Stir in the dried fruit bits and transfer to serving bowl. Allow to cool to room temperature. The pudding will turn a pale pink, thanks to the fruit. Very pretty. Garnish with mint. Even prettier.

GORGEOUS FRUIT CUSTARD
Four 1/2-cup servings

Spray vegetable oil
1 cup berries, fresh or frozen (blueberries? strawberries? raspberries?
    a mixture? your choice)
1/2 cup fat-free plain yogurt
1/2 cup fat-free cottage cheese
1/2 cup skim milk
1/4 cup egg substitute
1/4 cup flour
1/4 cup sugar
1 teaspoon vanilla extract

■ Preheat oven to 425°.
■ Lightly spray four 6-ounce custard cups and divide fruit equally among them. Put yogurt, cottage cheese, and milk into a blender and process until smooth. Add egg substitute and process again. Add flour, sugar, and vanilla and process once more. Pour over fruit and bake until golden brown and set, about 30 minutes.
■ The custard will sort of collapse a bit as it cools, but that's part of the dish. Not to worry.

**NOTES FOR
THE COOK:**
This shows how easily
you can transform
simple frozen fruit into
a delicious topping.

REAL FRUIT TOPPING
Two 1/2-cup servings

1 tablespoon corn starch
2 tablespoons water
2 cups whole frozen berries or mango, divided

■ Dissolve corn starch in water. Set aside. Cook 1 cup of the fruit until bubbly. Whisk until puréed. Add the dissolved corn starch and whisk until thickened. Add the remaining 1 cup of fruit and turn off the heat. This added fruit will remain whole in the thickened fruit puree. Serve over whole wheat waffle, pancakes, even whole grain toast.

**NOTES FOR
THE COOK:**
Cold morning? Want a
warm treat? This
takes apples to a new
level — and the house
will smell good, too.

APPLES BAKED IN BOILED CIDER
Four servings

4 cups apple cider
1/4 teaspoon ground cinnamon, optional
4 large Granny Smith apples, unpeeled, washed and cored
4 tablespoons raisins

■ Preheat oven to 350°.
■ Boil cider until reduced to 2 cups. Add cinnamon if desired. Put apples in baking dish, fill holes with raisins, and poke with sharp fork here and there to allow steam to escape through the skin. Pour cider over all. Bake until tender, about 50-60 minutes.

LUNCH

PERSONAL PIZZAS

Four servings

8 slices whole grain bread
1 package fat-free mozzarella (Kraft, for example)
3/4 cup Sun-dried Tomato Paste (recipe follows)

■ Broil bread on one side. Turn over and spread each slice with a heaping tablespoon of Sun-dried Tomato Paste. Divide the cheese 8 ways and sprinkle on pizza. Broil until cheese melts.

SUN-DRIED TOMATO PASTE

Makes about 3/4 cup

1 8-ounce jar sun-dried tomatoes marinated in olive oil, drained
1 scallion, coarsely chopped
Freshly ground pepper

■ Put the sun-dried tomatoes and scallion into food processor bowl. Add a generous dose of pepper. Process until smooth.

NOTES FOR THE COOK:
Experiment with different fat-free cheeses, and find one you like for its taste and meltability. By the way, you're getting a triple whammy: whole grain, vegetable, and low-fat dairy. Try this when the grandkids visit, too. They'll love it.

NOTES FOR THE COOK:
This makes a great spread — on a Personal Pizza, in a sandwich, or on a whole grain cracker.

NOTES FOR
THE COOK:
The salad can be used
as an appetizer, on a
sandwich, or piled on
greens for a real treat
This will look
somewhat unfamiliar,
maybe more like a
vegetable spread than
the creamy tuna salad
you might get at your
local sandwich shop.
But it is delicious and
you will be eating a lot
of vegetables!

THE BEST SALMON SALAD
Two servings

This calls for leftover salmon, which you will have because . . . you'll buy an extra 1/4 pound when you plan to cook salmon.

1/4 pound leftover cooked salmon
1 stalk of celery, finely chopped
1 small onion, finely chopped
1/4 red pepper, finely chopped
1 teaspoon mustard
1 tablespoon of ajvar or hot sauce
1 heaping tablespoon lite mayonnaise

■ Flake salmon. Mix in the chopped vegetables, mustard, hot sauce, and mayonnaise.

NOTES FOR
THE COOK:
Embarrassingly
simple and delicious,
this cold soup gives
you a chance to get a
lot of vegetables very
handily. We know a
woman who makes
gazpacho by putting
leftover salad,
dressing and all, into
the food processor
with V8 juice. She
swears by it. If an
actual recipe is more
your style, try this.

GAZPACHO
Makes three 1-cup servings

2 cups low sodium V8 juice
1/4 cup raw turnip, chopped
1/2 cup peeled, seeded, cucumber (about 1/2 medium cucumber), chopped
1/4 cup celery, chopped
1/4 cup yellow pepper, chopped
1/4 cup sweet onion, chopped
1/4 cup carrots, chopped
Freshly ground pepper to taste.

■ Put juice and vegetables into blender and process very briefly. Add pepper.

12 BEAN SOUP

(Don't worry! The beans come ready-mixed!)
About eight 1-cup servings

2 cups mixed dried beans (they come in 16-ounce packages)
6 cups water
1 large onion, chopped
3 celery stalks, chopped
1 red pepper, chopped
1 green pepper, chopped
3 cloves of garlic, minced
4 carrots, peeled and chopped
1 10-ounce package frozen cut green beans
1 large can low sodium V8 juice
1 14.5-ounce can diced tomatoes, no salt added
To taste:
Pepper, marjoram, thyme, and oregano

■ Soak beans overnight in water in a pot that is half-filled with water. Drain and rinse beans. Add 6 cups water. Bring to a boil, reduce heat, and simmer for about two hours or until beans are tender. While soup is simmering, sauté the onion, celery, peppers, and garlic. Add to beans. Add carrots and simmer until tender. Add green beans, V8 juice, and tomatoes. Simmer an additional 30 minutes.

NOTES FOR THE COOK:
Making a big pot of vegetable and bean soup every couple of weeks is a path to getting your vegetables. You will feel all cozy and productive with the cutting and stirring. And quite proud of the cache of ready-made meals stored in your freezer. Can be frozen in individual portions for great lunches — or invite the gang for dinner.

BONUS! BONUS!

A recipe to chuckle over — a soup to enjoy

BUTTERNUT SQUASH SOUP

Makes about 8 cups

2 tablespoons canola oil
1 large onion, chopped
1 large granny smith apple, peeled, cored, and sliced
3 medium butternut squash, peeled, seeded, and cubed
2 14.5-ounce cans chicken broth, fat free and low sodium
2 cups apple cider
Freshly ground pepper to taste

■ Heat oil in large stockpot. Add onion and apple. Sauté until softened and beginning to brown, about 5 minutes. Add squash and sauté for another 5 minutes.

■ Add broth and cider, bring mixture to boil, reduce heat to simmer, and cook, covered, until squash is very tender, about 20 minutes. Remove from heat and process in blender in batches. Add pepper and serve hot.

Alternate directions, by Deborah Levy

■ Heat oil in a large stockpot. Burn till smoke in kitchen is thick. Fan and air out (10 minutes). Scour pot.

■ Begin again. Heat oil in large stockpot. Add onion with force, splattering oil on forearms. Run arms under cold water (2 minutes). Sauté onion and apple until softened and beginning to brown, about 5 minutes. Add squash and sauté for another 5 minutes.

■ Forget you are cooking something for 12 minutes. Run back to stove, add broth and cider, and bring mixture to boil. Reduce heat to simmer and, if using a gas stove, accidentally extinguish flame. Read magazine for 10 minutes while expecting pot to boil.

■ Relight stove, bring mixture to boil again, reduce heat to simmer again, then cover and cook until squash is very tender, about 20 minutes. Remove from heat and process in blender in batches. On last batch, let blender top fly off, allowing soup to splatter all areas of kitchen and clothing. Add pepper. Serve hot.

■ **HOT TIP:** Allow soup to cool before processing in blender!

ENDNOTES

IN ORDER TO STUDY WHY PEOPLE DEVELOP DISEASE, researchers have been observing and analyzing data from thousands of people over long periods of time. We call this an epidemiological study. A group of people is selected; each individual reports to the researchers on a regular basis, fills in questionnaires, and possibly has a medical exam or sends medical records. These studies are designed to track the people in the study until the end of the story, called the "endpoint". In the case of each individual in an epidemiological study, the end of the story may be a disease (hospitalization, stroke, heart attack, cancer), or death. And then the researchers try to figure out if any "patterns" decrease the risk of those outcomes. Epidemiological studies point to important patterns that will need more thorough examination.

As an example, there was a time not so long ago in the history of scientific research when we did not know that high cholesterol levels meant you had a high risk of heart disease. Two important epidemiological studies, The Framingham Study in 1979 and MRFIT (Multiple Risk Factor Intervention Trial) in 1986, both showed that cholesterol levels predict heart disease. Researchers took this pattern and did more thorough research and proved that cholesterol is a risk factor in the development of heart disease. The rest is history.

We are making more history right now, as researchers observe patterns and find ways to improve health. For 55 years, epidemiological studies have shaped public health policy, and the work continues to this day.

This book is deeply grateful to the researchers and the participants in these studies:

☞ Iowa Women's Health Study: 34,492 postmenopausal woman (age 55 to 69) without heart disease (from Iowa).

☞ Nurses' Health Study: 68,782 woman from 37 to 64 years old without angina, myocardial infarction, stroke, cancer, high cholesterol or diabetes from all over the United States.

☞ Adventist Health Study: 34,198 White, non-Hispanic, Seventh Day Adventists from California (1988).

☞ Framingham Heart Study: 5,209 men and women between the ages of 30 and 62 from the town of Framingham, Massachusetts (1948) and in 1971, a second generation study of 5,124 of the original participants' adult children and their spouses.

These are the studies that back up THE BEST DIET ON EARTH, so that it can make the claim that ordinary foods have extraordinary powers

PATTERNS

IF YOU LOOK OVER all the great epidemiological studies of the last 55 years, you will see a pattern emerging: Eat more fruits and vegetables and whole grains and less saturated fat, and do more exercise. Clearly, it is not one food or one vitamin that will give you health. It is a pattern of foods.

The next step in scientific discovery is to take a "pattern" observed from the data and test whether this pattern holds true in a carefully controlled scientific experiment. This is called an" intervention study." The DASH diet has a special claim to fame because it was the first intervention study to examine a health response (changes in blood pressure) to a *pattern of eating*. DASH clearly showed that a *pattern of eating* was a powerful tool to lower blood pressure.

More and more, there is talk of patterns. If you look closely at the recommendations of all the major health organization in the United States, you will find a similar trend— a "unified approach" to healthy eating. This is just another way of saying "patterns." We are all talking about the same pattern. Patterns are so important that we have devoted a whole chapter to the topic.

■ Freeland-Graves J, Nitzke S. Position of the American Dietetic Association: Total Diet Approach to Communicating Food and Nutrition Information. *Journal of the American Dietetic Association.* 2002;102(1):100-108.

■ Dixon LB, Cronin FJ, Krebs-Smith SM. Let the Pyramid Guide Your Food Choices: Capturing the Total Diet Concept. *The Journal of Nutrition.* 2001;131(2S-1):461S-472S.

■ Nicklas TA, Baranowski T, Cullen KW, et al. Eating Patterns, Dietary Quality and Obesity. *Journal of the American College of Nutrition.* 2001;20(6):599-608.

■ Gillman MW, Rifas-Shiman SL, Frazier AL, et al. Family Dinner and Diet Quality Among Older Children and Adolescents. *Archives of Family Medicine.* 2000;9(3):235-240.

■ Deckelbaum RJ, Fisher EA, Winston M, et al. Summary of a Scientific Conference on Preventative Nutrition: Pediatrics to Geriatrics. *Circulation.* 1999;100:450-456.

WEIGHT LOSS

RESEARCHERS ARE BEGINNING TO UNDERSTAND how people lose weight, and, more importantly, how they keep it off. A group of scientists led by the esteemed F. Xavier Pi-Sunyer analyzed about 15 years of published research on weight loss. Their excellent conclusions are central to our understanding of how to achieve successful weight loss. See the Consensus Statement by the National Institute of Health.

But wait, what about real people, like you and me? Real people, who want to lose weight, and keep it off . . . but are not part of a research trial? For a wonderful understanding of how real people successfully maintain weight loss on their own (without being a part of a controlled study), read the research from The National Weight Control Registry (NWCR). Dr. James Hill and Dr. Rena Wing started this registry about 10 years ago to follow the weight loss patterns of real people. *http://www.uchsc.edu/ nutrition/nwcr.htm*

If you think you cannot lose weight, let's look at the information from the more than 2000 people who have joined the registry. Over the past five years, certain patterns are emerging about these "successful losers." They worked hard and made major changes in their diet and in their exercise program. Here are some of the findings:

☞ The average individual in the registry lost approximately 60 pounds and kept it off for about five years. This amount was about 30% of the pre-diet weight.

☞ Two-thirds of these people had a family history of obesity, and, moreover, were overweight when they were children.

☞ Approximately half the participants lost weight on their own, without the help of any kind of weight loss program.

☞ Here's an interesting finding in the people participating in this registry. Resting metabolism was similar in people of normal weight and in those who successfully lost weight.

Anyone can enroll in the NWCR, but in order to do so, you must have lost at least 30 pounds and kept it off for at least a year. There is no charge to enter (nor are you paid for participating), but you must be at least 18 years old. Your name will be kept confidential. While this registry is not a treatment program, you will join the club of successful losers. Join the losers! 1-800-606- NWCR (6927).

■ Smiciklas-Wright H, Mitchell DC, Mickle SJ, et al. Foods Commonly Eaten in the United States. Quantities Consumed Per Eating Occasion and in a Day, 1994-1996. United States Department of Agriculture NFS Report No. 96-5 pre-publication version, 252 pp. 2002. For internet information, visit: *www.barc.usda.gov/bhrnc/food survey/Products94961.html*

■ Astrup A, Grunwald GK, Melanson EL, et al. The Role of Low-Fat Diets in Body Weight Control: A Meta-Analysis of *Ad Libitum* Dietary Intervention Studies. *International Journal of Obesity.* 2000;(24):1545-1552

■ McGuire MT, Wing RR, Klem ML, et al. What Predicts Weight Regain in a Group of Successful Weight Losers? *Journal of Consulting and Clinical Psychology.* 1999;67(2):177-185.

■ McGuire MT, Wing RR, Klem ML, et al. Long-Term Maintenance of Weight Loss: Do People Who Lose Weight Through Various Weight Loss Methods Use Different Behaviors to Maintain Their Weight? *International Journal of Obesity.* 1998;(22):572-577.

■ National Institutes of Health, National Heart, Lung and Blood Institute. "Clinical Guidelines on the Identification, Evaluation, and Treatment of Overweight and Obesity in Adults: The Evidence Report 1998," *NIH Publication No. 98-4083.* Available at: *http://www.nhlbi.nih.gov/guidelines*

■ Shick SM, Wing RR, Klem ML, et al. Persons Successful at Long-Term Weight Loss and Maintenance Continue to Consume a Low-Energy, Low-Fat Diet. *Journal of the American Dietetic Association.* 1998;98(4):408-413.

■ Klem ML, Wing RR, McGuire MT, et al. A Descriptive Study of Individuals Successful at Long-Term Maintenance of Substantial Weight Loss. *American Journal of Clinical Nutrition.* 1997;66:239-246.

■ Fletcher AM. *Thin For Life: 10 keys to success from people who have lost weight and kept it off.* Houghton Mifflin Co., 1994.

BREAKFAST

A TRULY HEALTHY DAY starts with breakfast, so don't forget to eat it! Not only does eating breakfast improve your chances of getting all the vitamins, minerals, and phytochemicals you need to stay healthy, but it also increases the likelihood that you can keep a healthy weight. The National Weight Control Registry has shown that a person who eats breakfast regularly is more likely to be a successful loser.

■ Wyatt HR, Grunwald GK, Mosca CL, et al. Long-Term Weight Loss and Breakfast in Subjects in the National Weight Control Registry. *Obesity Research.* 2002;10(2):78-82.

■ Nicklas TA, Reger C, Myers L, et al. Breakfast Consumption With and Without Vitamin-Mineral Supplement Use Favorably Impacts Daily Nutrient Intake of Ninth-Grade Students. *Journal of Adolescent Health.* 2000;27(5):314-321.

■ Morgan KJ, Zabik ME, Stampley GL. The Role of Breakfast in Diet Adequacy of the U.S. Adult Population. *Journal of the American College of Nutrition.* 1986;5(6):551-563.

WHOLE GRAINS

WHOLE GRAINS CONTAIN ALL THE COMPONENTS of the grain: bran, germ, and starch. Each tiny individual kernel of grain is a "seed of life," and, when planted, supplies the nutrients for a whole new plant. These seeds are also important for our health. Whether we eat them whole (oats, corn, or barley) or ground (wheat or rye), we are getting the best food on earth. How do we know that? Compelling evidence indicates whole grains lower the risk of heart disease, cancer, and diabetes.

Several large studies — the Nurses Health Study, the Iowa Women's Health Study, and a Finnish study — have shown that people who eat whole grains have a lower risk of heart disease. Women in the Nurses Health study who ate whole grains were less likely to develop diabetes. We also have over 40 studies examining 20 different types of cancer that indicate whole grains reduce the risk of several types of cancers: stomach, colon, mouth, gallbladder, and ovaries.

■ Pereira MA, Jacobs Jr. DR, Pins JJ, et al. Effect of Whole Grains on Insulin Sensitivity in Overweight Hyperinsulinemic Adults. *American Journal of Clinical Nutrition*. 2002;75(5):848-855.

■ van Dam RM, Rimm EB, Willett WC, et al. Dietary Patterns and Risk for Type 2 Diabetes Mellitus in U.S. Men. *Annals of Internal Medicine*. 2002;136:201-209. *www.annals.org/issues/ v136n3/abs/ 200202050-00008.html*

■ Kantor LS, Variyam JN, Allshouse JE, et al. Choose a Variety of Grains Daily, Especially Whole Grains: A Challenge for Consumers. *The Journal of Nutrition*. 2001;131(2S-1):473S-486S.

■ Slavin JL, Jacobs D, Marquart L, et al. The Role Of Whole Grains In Disease Prevention. *Journal of the American Dietetic Association*. 2001;101(7):780-785.

■ Adams JF, Engstrom A. Helping Consumers Achieve Recommended Intakes of Whole Grain Foods. *Journal of the American College of Nutrition*. 2000;19(3):339S-344S.

■ Cleveland LE, Moshfegh AJ, Albertson AM, et al. Dietary Intake of Whole Grains. *Journal of the American College of Nutrition*. 2000;19(3):331S-338S.

■ Jacobs DR, Pereira MA, Meyer KA, et al. Fiber from Whole Grains, but Not Refined Grains, is Inversely Associated with All-Cause Mortality In Older Women: The Iowa Women's Health Study. *Journal of the American College of Nutrition*. 2000;19(3):326S-330S.

■ Liu S, Manson JE, Stampfer MJ, et al. A Prospective Study of Whole-Grain Intake and Risk of Type 2 Diabetes Mellitus in U.S. Women. *American Journal of Public Health*. 2000;90(9):1409-1415.

■ Liu S, Manson JE, Stampfer MJ, et al. Whole Grain Consumption and Risk of Ischemic Stroke in Women: A Prospective Study. *Journal of the American Medical Association*. 2000;284(12):1534-1540.

■ Jacobs DR, Meyer KA, Kushi LH, et al. Is Whole Grain Intake Associated with Reduced Total and Cause-Specific Death Rates in Older Women? The Iowa Women's Health Study. *American Journal of Public Health*. 1999;89(3):322-329.

■ Pietinen P, Rimm EB, Korhonen P, et al. Intake of Dietary Fiber and Risk of Coronary Heart Disease in a Cohort of Finnish Men. The Alpha-Tocopherol, Beta-Carotene Cancer Prevention Study. *Circulation*. 1996;94:2720-2727.

■ Welsh S, Shaw A, Davis C. Achieving Dietary Recommendations: Whole-Grain Foods in the Food Guide Pyramid. *Critical Reviews in Food Science and Nutrition*. 1994;34(5&6):441-451.

FRUITS AND VEGETABLES

WHAT'S OLD IS NEW AGAIN! Here is some new information about a very old-fashioned pattern of eating.

■ Ayoob KT, Duyff RL, Quagliani D. Position of the American Dietetic Association: Food and Nutrition Misinformation. *Journal of the American Dietetic Association*. 2002;102(2):260-266.

■ Joshipura KJ, Hu FB, Manson JE, et al. The Effect of Fruit and Vegetable Intake on Risk for Coronary Heart Disease. *Annals of Internal Medicine*. 2001;134(12):1106-1114.

■ Johnston CS, Taylor CA, Hampl JS. More Americans Are Eating "5 A Day," but Intakes of Dark Green and Cruciferous Vegetables Remain Low. *Journal of Nutrition*. 2000;130(12):3063-3067.

■ Rimm EB, Ascherio A, Giovannucci E, et al. Vegetable, Fruit, and Cereal Fiber Intake and Risk Of Coronary Heart Disease Among Men. *Journal of the American Medical Association*. 1996;275(6):447-451.

■ Krebs-Smith SM, Cook A, Subar AF, et al. U.S. Adults' Fruit and Vegetable Intakes, 1989 to 1991: A Revised Baseline for the Healthy People 2000 Objective. *American Journal of Public Health*. 1995;85(12):1623-1629.

EXERCISE

YOU ALREADY KNOW you are supposed to exercise. And you want to, really you do, don't you? You know it's good for you. You hear the message. Now there are new government guidelines that have raised the "30-minutes-most-days" bar. The new gold standard is ONE HOUR OF PHYSICAL ACTIVITY EVERY DAY. For advanced reading about exercise check out these fancy reports. All are available on the web at *http://www.acsm-msse.org/*

☞ The Recommended Quantity and Quality of Exercise for Developing and Maintaining Cardiorespiratory and Muscular Fitness, and Flexibility in Healthy Adults.

☞ Exercise and Physical Activity for Older Adults.

☞ Exercise and Type 2 Diabetes.

Another web site devoted to helping us get our exercise act together is the Shape Up America web site: *http://www.shapeup.org/publications/fitting.fitness.in/noframes/topreasons.htm*

But how to get enough exercise? *The Best Diet on Earth* suggests using legs and a sidewalk. Plus a handy little tool called a pedometer to keep you on track, remind you to walk more, and make walking a challenge for excellence. Only recently have we begun to see research that demonstrates a pedometer can be an effective health aid. Here are some nice little studies that pave the way for more widespread acceptance of the "step way" to exercise.

■ Diabetes Prevention Program Research Group. Reduction in the Incidence of Type 2 Diabetes with Lifestyle Intervention or Metformin. *New England Journal of Medicine*. 2002;346(6):393-403.

■ Iwane M, Arita M,Tomimoto S, et al. Walking 10,000 Steps/Day or More Reduces Blood Pressure and Sympathetic Nerve Activity in Mild Essential Hypertension. *Hypertension Research*. 2000;23(6):573-580.

■ Manson JE, Greenland PG, LaCroix AZ, et al. Walking Compared with Vigorous Exercise for the Prevention of Cardiovascular Events in Women. *New England Journal of Medicine*. 2002;347(10):716-725.

▓ Sugiura H, Sugiura H, Kajima K, et al. Effects of Long-Term Moderate Exercise and Increase in Number of Daily Steps on Serum Lipids in Women: Randomized Controlled Trial. *BMC Women's Health*.2002; 2(3): 1-8.

▓ Tudor-Locke C. Taking Steps Toward Increased Physical Activity: Using Pedometers to Measure and Motivate. President's Council on Physical Fitness and Sports. *Research Digest*. 2002;3(17):1-8.

▓ Tudor-Locke CE, Bell RC, Myers AM, et al. Pedometer-Determined Ambulatory Activity in Individuals with Type 2 Diabetes. *Diabetes Research and Clinical Practice*. 2002;55(3):191-199.

▓ Moreau KL, Degarmo R, Langley J, et al. Increasing Daily Walking Lowers Blood Pressure in Postmenopausal Women. *Medicine & Science in Sports & Exercise*. 2001;33(11):1825-1831.

▓ Speck BJ, Looney SW. Effects of a Minimal Intervention to Increase Physical Activity in Women: Daily Activity Records. *Nursing Research*. 2001;50(6):374-378.

▓ Tudor-Locke C, Ainsworth BE, Whitt MC, et al. The Relationship Between Pedometer-Determined Ambulatory Activity and Body Composition Variables. *International Journal of Obesity*. 2001; 25(11):1571-1578.

▓ Bassett DR, Ainsworth BE, Leggett SR, et al. Accuracy of Five Electronic Pedometers for Measuring Distance Walked. *Medicine & Science in Sports & Exercise* 1996;28(8):1071-1077.

▓ Yamanouchi K, Shinozaki T, Chikada K, et al. Daily Walking Combined with Diet Therapy is a Useful Means for Obese NIDDM Not Only to Reduce Body Weight, but also to Improve Insulin Sensitivity. *Diabetes Care*. 1995;18:775-778.

DASH STUDY RESULTS

A FEW MORE WORDS OF ADMIRATION: The DASH study is a state-of-the-art intervention study. And it was the first large-scale U.S. trial to assess specific dietary patterns using commonly available foods. The results are impressive: The level of blood pressure reductions was far greater than observed in any prior nutrition study and equals those attainable with drug treatment. The DASH diet controlled BP in 70% of the people who had Stage 1 hypertension. (Systolic BP > or equal to 140 mm Hg and/or Diastolic greater than or equal to 90 mm Hg.) Not only that, but people loved to be a part of the study, with an amazing adherence for all groups (control, fruit and vegetable, and combination). Completion of the study in the combination group was 98.7%! Attendance at on-site meal locations was 96.1%! Check out these articles:

▓ Obarzanek E, Sacks FM, Vollmer WM, et al. DASH Research Group; Effects on Blood Lipids of a Blood Pressure-Lowering Diet: The Dietary Approaches to Stop Hypertension (DASH) Trial. *American Journal of Clinical Nutrition*. 2001;74(1):80-89.

■ Appel LJ, Miller III ER, Ha Jee S, et al. Effect of Dietary Patterns on Serum Homocysteine: Results of a Randomized, Controlled Feeding Study. *Circulation*. 2000;102:852-857.

■ Conlin PR, Chow D, Miller III ER, et al. The Effect Of Dietary Patterns on Blood Pressure Control in Hypertensive Patients: Results from the Dietary Approaches To Stop Hypertension (DASH) Trial. *American Journal of Hypertension*. 2000;13:949-955.

■ Harsha DW, Lin PH, Obarzanek E, et al. Dietary Approaches to Stop Hypertension: A Summary of Study Results. *Journal of The American Dietetic Association*.1999;99(8):S35-S39.

■ Karanja NM, Obarzanek E, Lin PH, et al. Descriptive Characteristics of the Dietary Patterns Used in the Dietary Approaches to Stop Hypertension Trial. *Journal of The American Dietetic Association*. 1999;99(8):SI9-S27.

■ Plaisted CS, Lin PH, Ard JD, et al. The Effects of Dietary Patterns on Quality of Life: A substudy of The Dietary Approaches to Stop Hypertension Trial. *Journal of The American Dietetic Association*.1999;99(8):S84-S89.

■ Vogt TM, Appel LJ, Obarzanek E, et al. Dietary Approaches to Stop Hypertension: Rationale, Design, and Methods. *Journal of The American Dietetic Association*. 1999;99(8):S12-S18.

■ Windhauser MM, Evans MA, McCullough ML, et al. Dietary Adherence in the Dietary Approaches to Stop Hypertension Trial. *Journal of The American Dietetic Association*. 1999;99(8):S76-S83.

■ Windhauser MM, Ernst DB, Karanja NM, et al. Translating the Dietary Approaches to Stop Hypertension Diet from Research to Practice: Dietary and Behavior Change Techniques. *Journal of The American Dietetic Association*. 1999;99(8):S90-S95.

■ National Institute of Health, National Heart, Lung and Blood Institute. Facts About The DASH Diet. Bethesda, Md.1998. *NIH Publication No. 98-4082. http://www.nhlbi.nih.gov/ health/public/heart/hbp/ dash/*

■ Appel LJ, Moore TJ, Obarzanek E, et al. A Clinical Trial of the Effects of Dietary Patterns on Blood Pressure: DASH Collaborative Research Group. *New England Journal of Medicine*. 1997;336:1117-1124.

DASH & SODIUM; LOWERING SODIUM EVEN MORE...

■ Sacks FM, Svetkey LP, Vollmer VM, et al. Effects on Blood Pressure of Reduced Dietary Sodium and the Dietary Approaches to Stop Hypertension (DASH) Diet. *New England Journal Of Medicine*. 2001;344(1):3-10.

FISH

FISH IS ANOTHER PART OF THE BEST DIET ON EARTH. Eating fish at least once a week offers protection from sudden cardiac death.

■ Hu FB, Bronner L, Willett WC, et al. Fish and Omega-3 Fatty Acid Intake and Risk of Coronary Heart Disease in Women. *Journal of the American Medical Association.* 2002; 287(14):1815-1821.

■ Albert CM, Hennekens CH, O'Donnell CJ, et al. Fish Consumption and Risk of Sudden Cardiac Death. *Journal of the American Medical Association.* 1998;279(1):23-28.

MEAT

ARE YOU AFRAID TO EAT RED MEAT? Some highly regarded researchers have demonstrated that lean red meat is just as good for your cholesterol as "whiter" meat, such as chicken, pork, and veal. Of course, the size of the serving should more closely resemble a deck of cards than a placemat.

■ Hunninghake DB, Maki KC, Kwiterovich PO, et al. Incorporation of Lean Red Meat into a National Cholesterol Education Program Step I Diet: A Long-Term, Randomized Clinical Trial In Free-Living Persons With Hypercholesterolemia. *Journal of the American College of Nutrition.* 2000;19(3):351-360.

■ Davidson MH, Hunninghake D, Maki KC, et al. Comparison of the Effects of Lean Red Meat vs. Lean White Meat on Serum Lipid Levels Among Free-Living Persons with Hypercholesterolemia. *Archives of Internal Medicine.* 1999;159:1331-1338.

MILK

MOM WAS RIGHT. Drink your milk.

■ Zemel MB. Mechanisms of Dairy Modulation of Adiposity. *Journal of Nutrition.* 2003; 133(1): 252S-256S.

■ Pereira MA, Jacobs DR, Van Horn L, et al. Dairy Consumption, Obesity, and the Insulin Resistance Syndrome in Young Adults. The CARDIA Study. *Journal of the American Medical Association.* 2002;287(16):2081-2089.

■ Hjartaker A, Laake P, Lund E. Childhood and Adult Milk Consumption and Risk Of Premenopausal Breast Cancer in a Cohort of 48,844 Women — The Norwegian Women and Cancer Study. *International Journal of Cancer.* 2001;93(6):888-893.

■ Miller GD, DiRienzo DD, Reusser ME, et al. Benefits of Dairy Product Consumption on Blood Pressure in Humans: A Summary of the Biomedical Literature. *Journal of the American College of Nutrition.* 2000;19(2):147S-164S.

■ McBean LD, Miller GD. Allaying Fears and Fallacies about Lactose Intolerance. *Journal of the American Dietetic Association.*1998;98:671-676.

NUTS

IT'S A PLEASURE TO TELL PEOPLE to include nuts in their food patterns, because nuts are a real treat! Walnuts, peanuts, almonds and other nuts have all been shown to be a part of a health protective food pattern and really should have a place of honor in the food pyramid.

So just what is it about the humble nut? Nuts are loaded with little miracle workers called phytochemicals and the plant fats that are heart protective. This "nut effect" was evident in The Adventist Health study, The Iowa Women's Health Study, The Nurses' Health Study, and the Physicians' Health Study. How many nuts? The jury is still out. The people who had the greatest reduction in heart events ate nuts frequently during the week— 4 to 5 times a week. About a one ounce serving of nuts is not unreasonable. An entire can of nuts, however, definitely is.

Type of Nut	How many nuts in an ounce?
Almonds	22 whole
Cashews	18 whole
Macadamia	10-12
Mixed nuts	10 nuts
Peanuts	33
Pecans	20 halves
Walnuts	14 halves

If you are worried about weight gain, you should know that it did not appear to be an issue in any of these studies. People who ate nuts gained no more weight than people who did not eat nuts. Just remember to keep an eye on serving size! Serving size is the key to the Healthy Weigh.

■ Albert CM, Gaziano JM, Willett WC, Manson JE. Nut Consumption and Decreased Risk of Sudden Cardiac Death in the Physicians' Health Study. *Archives of Internal Medicine*. 2002; 162(12): 1382-1387.

■ Feldman EB. The Scientific Evidence for a Beneficial Health Relationship Between Walnuts and Coronary Heart Disease. *The Journal of Nutrition*. 2002;132(5):1062S-1101S.

■ U.S. Department of Agriculture, Agricultural Research Service. 2002. USDA Nutrient Database for Standard Reference, Release 15. Nutrient Data Laboratory Home Page, *http://www.nal.usda.gov/fnic/ foodcomp*

■ Fraser GE. Nut Consumption, Lipids, and the Risk of a Coronary Event. *Clinical Cardiology*. 1999;22(Supp. III):11-15.

■ Hu FB, Stampfer MJ. Nut Consumption and Risk of Coronary Heart Disease: A Review of Epidemiological Evidence. *Current Atherosclerosis Reports*. 1999;1(3):204-209.

THE COST OF NOT FOLLOWING THE BEST DIET ON EARTH

IT IS GETTING VERY EXPENSIVE not to follow THE BEST DIET ON EARTH. In the United States, healthcare spending on the chronic medical conditions associated with obesity is greater than the healthcare spending on conditions resulting from smoking.

Now for some good news: The cost of eating fruits, vegetables, whole grains, and dairy is about the amount the average American spends each week on groceries. Believe it or not, our government keeps track of what we spend on food. And the verdict is in: You **CAN** afford to follow THE BEST DIET ON EARTH.

▓ "Consumers' Expenditures in 2000," *US Dept of Labor, Bureau of Labor Statistics*, April 2002. Report 958. Available at: *http://www.bls.gov/cex/csxann00.pdf*

▓ "Official USDA Food Plans: Cost of Food at Home at Four Levels, US Average April 2002." *United States Department of Agriculture, Center for Policy and Promotion.* (Family of two: $60 to $115 dollars per week for food. This type of USDA information was used to make sure that the foods for DASH fit the average food costs in US. For other family models, see report.) *Available at: http://www.usda.gov/cnpp/ FoodPlans/Updates/foodfapr02.pdf*

▓ Sturm R.The Effects of Obesity, Smoking, and Drinking on Medical Problems and Costs. *Health Affairs.* 2002;21(1):245-253.

TRANS FAT

TRANS FAT ACTS LIKE SATURATED FAT IN THE BODY — raising cholesterol levels and increasing the risk of heart disease. Our government recognizes the health dangers of trans fat, so soon you will be seeing it on the Nutrition Facts Label (appropriately included as part of Saturated Fat.)

But if you are eating THE BEST DIET ON EARTH, you will have little chance of getting this unhealthy fat, since most of the trans fat in American diets is found in baked products. So eat the whole foods in THE BEST DIET ON EARTH and forget about trans fat.

▓ Oomen CM, Ocké MC, Feskens EJ, et al. Association between Trans Fatty Acid Intake and 10-Year Risk Of Coronary Heart Disease in the Zutphen Elderly Study: A Prospective Population-Based Study. *Lancet.* 2001;357(9258):746-751.

▓ Lichtenstein AH, Ausman LM, Jalbert SM, et al. Effects of Different Forms of Dietary Hydrogenated Fats on Serum Lipoprotein Cholesterol Levels. [published erratum appears in *New England Journal of Medicine.* 1999;341:856]. *New England Journal of Medicine.*1999;340:1933-1940.

SNACKING PATTERNS

EVERYTHING ABOUT THE SNACKING INDUSTRY IS BIG — it's big business, it makes big money, and it creates big people. Do your part to make American leaner: Choose healthy snacks.

■ Bell EA, Rolls BJ. Energy Density of Foods Affects Energy Intake Across Multiple Levels of Fat Content in Lean and Obese Women. *American Journal of Clinical Nutrition*. 2001;73:1010-1018.

■ Rolls BJ, Barnett RA. *Volumetrics*. New York: Harper Collins; 2000.

■ Rolls BJ, Bell EA, Castellanos VH, et al. Energy Density but Not Fat Content of Foods Affected Energy Intake in Lean and Obese Women. *American Journal of Clinical Nutrition*. 1999;69:863-871.

■ Rolls BJ, Bell EA. Intake of Fat and Carbohydrate: Role of Energy Density. *European Journal of Clinical Nutrition*. 1999;53(1):S166-S173.

TOXIC FOOD ENVIRONMENT

IT SEEMS AS IF EVERYTHING IS AGAINST YOU in your effort to eat a healthy diet. Not only is there so much prepared and fast food that is loaded with fat and calories, but serving sizes have grown to absurd proportions. A toxic environment indeed.

Some things are out of your control. When you live in a toxic environment, it is hard to make healthy choices.

■ Nestle M. *Food Politics: How the Food Industry Influences Nutrition and Health*. Berkeley: University of California Press; 2002.

■ Young LR, Nestle M. Contribution of Expanding Portion Sizes to the US Obesity Epidemic. *American Journal of Public Health*. 2002;92:246-249.

■ Zizza C, Siega-Riz AM, Popkin BM. Significant Increase in Young Adults' Snacking between 1977-1978 and 1994-1996 Represents a Cause for Concern! *Preventative Medicine*. 2001;32(4):303-310.

PROTECTING THE HEART

FOR THE MOST UP TO DATE INFORMATION on dealing with heart disease, see the following.

■ Thorand B, Lowel H, Schneider A, et al. C-Reactive Protein as a Predictor for Incident Diabetes Mellitus Among Middle-aged Men: Results From the MONICA Augsburg Cohort Study, 1984-1998. *Archives of Internal Medicine*. 2003; 163(1):93-99.

■ Hu FB, Willett WC. Optimal Diets for Prevention of Coronary Heart Disease. *Journal of the American Medical Association*. 2002; 288(20): 2569-2578.

■ Libby P, Ridker PM, Maseri A. Inflammation and Atherosclerosis. *Circulation*. 2002;105:1135.

■ Third report of the expert panel on detection, evaluation, and treatment of high blood cholesterol in adults (adult treatment panel III). National Heart, Lung, and Blood Institute web site. Available at: *http://www.nhlbi.nih.gov/guidelines/cholesterol/atp3_rpt.htm.*

■ Executive Summary of the Third Report of the National Cholesterol Education Program (NCEP) Expert Panel on Detection, Evaluation, and Treatment of High Blood Cholesterol in Adults (Adult Treatment Panel III). *Journal of the American Medical Association.* 2001;285:2486-2497.

INDEX